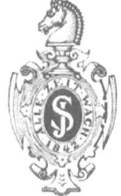

Recent Results in Cancer Research

Fortschritte der Krebsforschung

Progrès dans les recherches sur le cancer

11

Edited by

V. G. Allfrey, New York · M. Allgöwer, Chur · K. H. Bauer, Heidelberg · I. Berenblum, Rehovoth · F. Bergel, Jersey, C. I. · J. Bernard, Paris · W. Bernhard, Villejuif N. N. Blokhin, Moskva · H. E. Bock, Tübingen · P. Bucalossi, Milano · A. V. Chaklin, Moskva · M. Chorazy, Gliwice · G. J. Cunningham, London · W. Dameshek, Boston M. Dargent, Lyon · G. Della Porta, Milano · P. Denoix, Villejuif · R. Dulbecco, San Diego · H. Eagle, New York · R. Eker, Oslo · P. Grabar, Paris · H. Hamperl, Bonn R. J. C. Harris, London · E. Hecker, Heidelberg · R. Herbeuval, Nancy · J. Higginson, Lyon · W. C. Hueper, Bethesda · H. Isliker, Lausanne · D. A. Karnofsky, New York · J. Kieler, København · G. Klein, Stockholm · H. Koprowski, Philadelphia · L. G. Koss, New York · G. Martz, Zürich · G. Mathé, Paris · O. Mühlbock, Amsterdam · W. Nakahara, Tokyo · G. T. Pack, New York · V. R. Potter, Madison · A. B. Sabin, Cincinnati · L. Sachs, Rehovoth · E. A. Saxén, Helsinki W. Szybalski, Madison · H. Tagnon, Bruxelles · R. M. Taylor, Toronto · A. Tissières, Genève · E. Uehlinger, Zürich · R. W. Wissler, Chicago · T. Yoshida, Tokyo

Editor in chief
P. Rentchnick, Genève

Springer-Verlag Berlin Heidelberg New York 1967

Treatment of Skin Cancer

Robert G. Freeman · John M. Knox

With 32 Figures

Springer-Verlag Berlin Heidelberg New York 1967

Robert G. Freeman, M. D. (Glen), Associate Professor of Pathology and Dermatology, Baylor University College of Medicine, Houston, Texas/USA

John M. Knox, M. D., Professor and Chairman, Department of Dermatology, Baylor University College of Medicine, Houston, Texas/USA

Sponsored by the Swiss League against Cancer

ISBN 978-3-642-48251-9   ISBN 978-3-642-48249-6 (eBook)
DOI 10.1007/978-3-642-48249-6

Softcover reprint of the hard cover 1st edition 1967

Table of Contents

Introduction

Although skin cancer is the most common form of cancer and presents a consistent problem in recognition, in treatment, and in prevention, it usually does not receive as much attention as other more deadly forms of cancer. Nonetheless, a great deal of progress has been made toward understanding its cause and biological behavior as well as toward recognizing and treating early cancerous and pre-cancerous lesions. Today's physicians are more aware of early lesions and patients are seeking their advice on many small skin blemishes. In addition, clinicians are exploring new modalities of treatment, including chemotherapy. Some of these methods are very simple and effective for eradicating early lesions, and we are rapidly approaching the time in which the only reasons for a death due to skin cancer will be lack of a patient's cooperation or a physician's error in management.

The most important factors in improving the cure rate of skin cancer are a thorough knowledge of its cause and biological behavior and an understanding of the limitations of each modality of treatment.

The procedures and results outlined in this monograph record the experience of a large skin tumor service in the Baylor Affiliated Hospitals, but primarily at a charity hospital treating indigent patients, a group that tend to be less alert and less cooperative in matters of prevention and early treatment. The study covers a 15-year period of continuous operation and represents what can be accomplished under ordinary, perhaps less than optimal, conditions. The techniques used require no great expenditure of time, special equipment or great skill. They should be adaptable to most medical clinics.

Chapter 1

Etiology

Even though the cellular mechanisms whereby any cancer develops are not yet understood, a great deal is known about the circumstances and factors that predispose a person to skin cancer. The skin is exposed to the environment more than any other tissue of the body; thus environmental factors are more significant in skin cancer than in internal cancer. Although external physical insults are the major factors involved in the development of skin cancer, internally-administered agents and genetic background also are significant in some cases.

UNNA is credited as the first physician to emphasize the association of sun exposure and skin cancer by his description of "sailor's skin" [1], though archeological and historical records of costumes and daily habits of ancient peoples indicate that they were aware of the danger of sun exposure. Many of these customs persist today.

It is common knowledge that skin cancer is most prevalent among outdoor workers who have daily prolonged exposure to the sun. Even in the time of DUBREUILH, workers in the vineyards of Bordeaux had more skin cancer than their fellow man [2]. Also it is generally accepted that skin cancer usually develops on exposed areas of the body, and that it is more prevalent in regions of the world receiving intense sunlight [3]. The data of DORN reveal that the incidence of skin cancer increases as the latitude approaches the equator [4]. This latitude difference is paramount but is not the only factor contributing to an increase in the amount of sunlight exposure. Another factor is the obliqueness or directness of the pathway of sunlight through the atmosphere. The shortest and most direct pathway allowing the greatest penetration of light is when the sun is directly overhead, for example in tropical zones. At the equator there are also more hours per day in which intense sunlight hits the earth's surface. Local weather conditions are important, for example the number of cloudy days or the number of days during which inclement weather restricts outdoor activities.

In northern latitudes, light travels a more oblique path. Therefore it travels a longer distance through the atmosphere and there is atmospheric attenuation of all wavelengths. The shorter wavelengths, including harmful mid-ultraviolet, are filtered selectively by the ozone of the atmosphere and this selective filtration is accentuated when the pathways through the atmosphere are oblique. This phenomenon also decreases the ultraviolet content of early morning and late afternoon sunlight and results in less damaging exposure at these times.

Personal habits also enter into the question of sun exposure. For example some people habitually wear large hats and protective clothing while others are fadist sun bathers and outdoor worshipers [5].

Clinical and epidemiologic evidence of the relationship between sunlight exposure an skin cancer is supported by the work of FINDLEY [6−8], who experimentally produced skin cancer in mice by repeated ultraviolet exposure. ROFFO [9, 10] induced skin cancer in rats by exposing them to natural sunlight. He also blocked carcinogenesis by filtering sunlight through ordinary window glass. This indicated that the carcinogenic wavelengths were shorter than 3200 Å, the point below which glass filters out light. Since the shortest wavelength of sunlight reaching the earth's surface is approximately 2900 Å, the carcinogenic wavelengths in sunlight must then lie between 2900 and 3200 Å. Wavelengths shorter than 2900 Å are carcinogenic experimentally and while not of importance in human cancer today, may be important to future space travelers.

Another factor that accentuates ultraviolet injury of skin is heat. We have demonstrated that heat enhances ultraviolet carcinogenesis in mice. It also accentuates the erythemal effect of the ultraviolet light on human skin and possibly also the carcinogenic effect in man [11].

Most adult men in the Southwest areas of the United States have a sharp line of demarcation between exposed and unexposed skin such as at the collar line and wrists (Fig. 1). This demarcation is less noticeable in women, particularly in those who wear makeup regularly and avoid the intense mid-day sun. The phenomenon is more exaggerated in blonde, blue-eyed, fair-complexioned individuals and this correlates with their higher incidence of skin cancer. Dark-complexioned persons have fewer skin cancers. In fact, Negroes rarely develop actinically-induced cancer.

In a histologic study of men and women volunteers of different ages and different races, Negro skin showed no actinic degeneration. Rete ridges were preserved, even in elderly Negroes. By contrast we surprisingly found in young Caucasian adults, those in their 20's, extensive actinic degeneration of collagen as well as effacement of the rete ridges of the epidermis in exposed areas [12, 13]. This degeneration, the result of cumulative exposure, is considered permanent. However, transplantation of actinically damaged skin to protected sites allowed some regression of the degeneration, implying that the damage may be reversible in part [14].

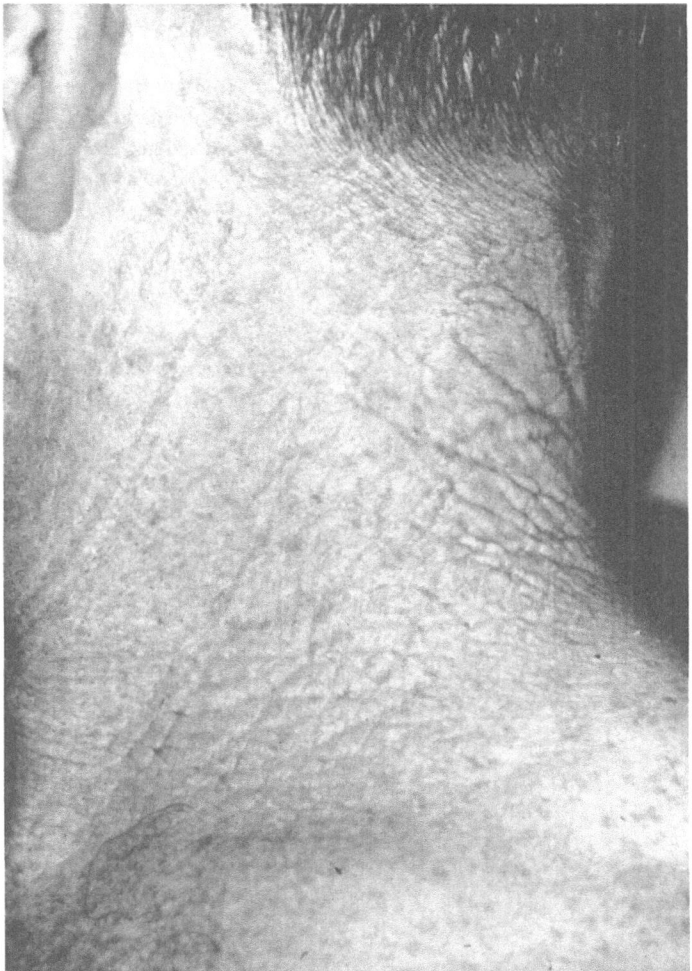

Fig. 1. Degeneration, wrinkling, and mottling of sun-damaged skin is limited to exposed areas with sharp demarcation as shown at the collar line in this 49 year old man

Actinic damage and the ultimate emergence of cancer is a result of chronic cumulative exposure to the mid-ultraviolet wavelengths of sunlight. We should remember that this chronic cumulative exposure begins in infancy and often is already well developed by adulthood.

While sunlight exposure is the paramount cause of most skin cancers, other factors must not be ignored. The frequent development of squamous cell carcinoma in an old burn scar (Marjolin's ulcer) is well known.

Unless the need makes it mandatory, roentgen therapy on exposed skin should be avoided in young people because they run a high risk of developing skin cancer in the irradiated area several decades later. We have already mentioned the genetic factor of complexion and skin color. An extreme example of genetic sensitivity to sunlight is seen in patients with xeroderma pigmentosa. Their inevitable course is skin cancers, malignant melanomas and an early death. The basal cell nevus syndrome in which multiple basal cell epitheliomas are associated with a variety of other congenital abnormalities also is transferred genetically [15].

As long ago as 1887, it was recognized that arsenic could be related etiologically to skin cancer [16]. Since then, even in the last decade, considerable evidence has been accumulated to show that arsenic is carcinogenic. This evidence indicates that arsenic is capable of producing the classical type of arsenical keratoses and cancers and that, in addition, it very likely is etiologically related to Bowen's disease and possibly other cutaneous and visceral cancers [17]. Notably FIERZ [18] found a 40 per cent incidence of hyperkeratosis palmaris et plantaris and 8 per cent skin cancer in 262 patients who had received arsenic as diluted Fowler's solution. He found both basal and squamous cancers, precancers and Bowen's disease. In addition to palmar and plantar localization, features suggesting arsenical etiology were onset at a young age, localization on the arms and trunk, multiplicity of lesions, and history of arsenic ingestion.

References

[1] UNNA, P. G.: Die Histopathologie der Hautkrankheiten. Berlin: A. Hirschewald 1894.
[2] DUBREUILH, W.: Ann. dermatologie syphilographie 8 (series 4), 387 (1907).
[3] BLUM, H. F.: Carcinogenesis by ultraviolet light. Princeton University Press: 1959, pp. 285—286.
[4] DORN, H. F.: Illness from cancer in the United States. Publ. Hlth Rep. 59, 33—48, 65—77, 97—115 (1944).
[5] MACDONALD, E. J.: The epidermilogy of skin cancer. J. invest. Derm. 32, 379—382 (1959).
[6] FINDLAY, G. M.: Ultra-violet light and skin cancer. Lancet 215, 1070 (1928).
[7] PUTSCHAR, M., and F. HOLTZ: Erzeugung von Hautkrebsen bei Ratten durch langdauernde Ultraviolettbestrahlung. Z. Krebsforsch. 33, 218 (1930).
[8] HERLITZ, C. W., I. JUNDELL, and F. WAHLGREN: Durch Ultraviolettbestrahlung erzeugte maligne Neubildungen bei weißen Mäusen. Acta Paediat. 10, 321 (1931).
[9] ROFFO, A. H.: Cancer et soleil. Carcinomes et sarcomes provoqués par l'action du soleil in toto. Bull. Ass. franç. Cancer 23, 590—616 (1934).
[10] FUNDING, G., O. M. HENRIQUES, and E. REKLING: Über Lichtkanzer. Dritter Internationaler Kongreß für Lichtforschung. Wiesbaden, 1936, pp. 166—168.
[11] FREEMAN, R. G., and J. M. KNOX: Influence of temperature on ultraviolet injury. Arch. Dermat. 89, 858—864 (1964).
[12] COCKERELL, E. G., R. G. FREEMAN, and J. M. KNOX: Changes after prolonged exposure to sunlight. Arch. Dermat. 84, 467—472 (1961).
[13] FREEMAN, R. G., E. G. COCKERELL, J. ARMSTRONG, and J. M. KNOX: Sunlight as a factor influencing the thickness of epidermis. J. invest. Derm. 39, 295—298 (1962).

[14] GERSTEIN, W., and R. G. FREEMAN: Transplantation of actinically damaged skin. J. invest. Derm. 41, 445—449 (1963).
[15] ANDERSON, D. E., J. L. McCLENDON, and J. B. HOWELL: Genetics and skin tumors with special reference to basal cell nevi. In Tumors of the skin. Chicago: Year Book Publishers, Inc. 1964, p. 91.
[16] HUTCHINSON, J.: Arsenic cancer. Brit. med. J. 2, 1280 (1887).
[17] GRAHAM, J. H., G. R. MAZZANTI, and E. B. HELWIG: Chemistry of Bowen's disease: Relationship to arsenic. J. invest. Derm. 37, 317 (1961).
[18] FIERZ, U.: Katamnestische Untersuchungen über die Nebenwirkungen der Therapie mit anorganischem Arsen bei Hautkrankheiten. Dermatologica 131, 41 (1965).

Chapter 2

Recognition and Diagnosis

Most failures in treatment of skin cancer can be traced to a mistake in the initial evaluation. Therefore the first important step is careful and thorough examination of the tumor. Great care should be given to determine what type the cancer is, how large it has grown, and if it has spread. This knowledge is essential to select the most appropriate method of treatment.

Physicians experienced in diagnosing and treating skin cancers can readily identify most skin cancers quite accurately by clinical examination alone. In a study of 3000 consecutive skin tumors treated by dermatologists in private practice, their accuracy in clinical diagnosis of all tumor types averaged 85 per cent [1]. There was some variation in accuracy with specific tumors. For example basal cell epitheliomas were recognized correctly 90 per cent of the time, while malignant melanomas were recognized correctly only 65 per cent of the time. When thorough examination has been combined with careful histopathologic study the chance for an accurate diagnosis is even higher—approaching 100 per cent. Thus to provide the greatest opportunity for accurate assessment and cure, pathologic diagnosis must accompany clinical diagnosis.

Most skin malignancies are either squamous cell carcinoma or basal cell epithelioma. The number of malignant melanomas and sarcomas is much smaller. In a recent five-year period in our pathology laboratory, 4,950 skin malignancies were submitted for diagnosis. Of this number, 3,709 were basal cell epitheliomas, 1,179 squamous cell carcinomas, 59 malignant melanomas and 3 sarcomas. Thus, all but 62 of the malignancies were either basal cell epithelioma or squamous cell carcinoma.

The ratio of basal to squamous tumors, approximately 3 to 1, is fairly representative for our geographic area. Surveys in geographic areas where sun exposure was low have shown a greater preponderance of basal cell epitheliomas. This change in the ratio correlates well with the variation in sunlight exposure in different geographic areas. It also indicates that while basal cell epitheliomas do occur on exposed areas and are related to sun exposure they require less energy for their production and their incidence does not correlate with sun exposure as closely as does the incidence of squamous cell carcinoma.

Squamous Cell Carinoma

Most squamous cell carcinomas we have encountered represent malignant transformation in an actinic keratosis—a premalignant condition. These tumors are found only on exposed areas, most commonly on the head, neck, hands and forearms. They first appear in areas of actinically degenerated skin as small, scaly, slightly

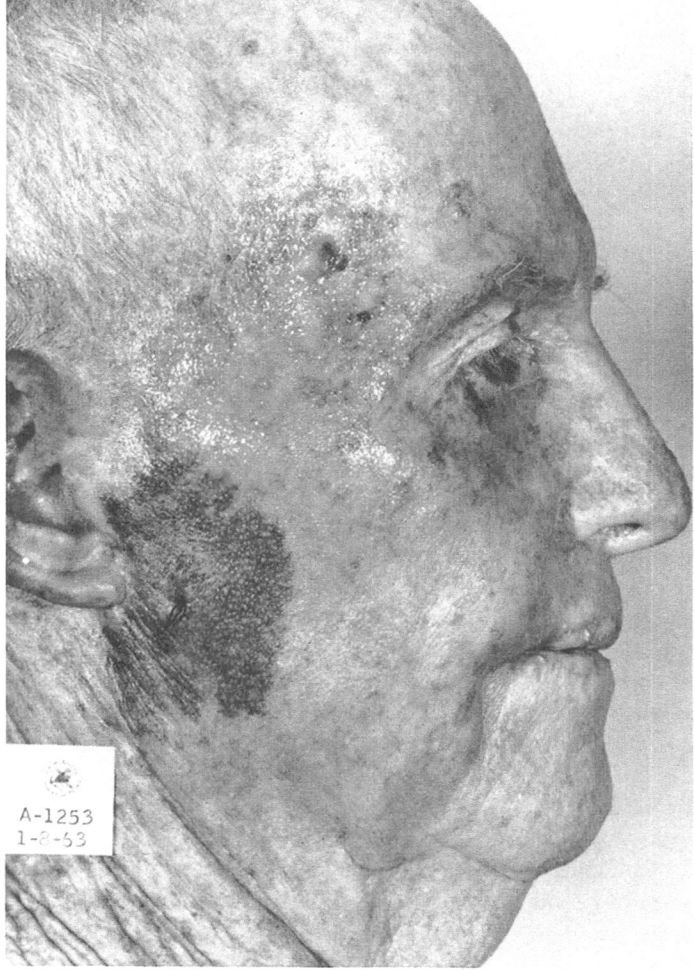

Fig. 2. This man manifests severe actinic degeneration and has multiple actinic keratoses. The dark preauricular lesion was biopsied and the diagnoses was intraepidermal squamous cell carcinoma

erythematous macules which can be recognized readily and treated easily with a variety of simple procedures (Figs. 2, 3, 4). Many patients will have several of these lesions; some may have a dozen or more. In older, more susceptible patients these lesions continue to appear. It is customary for these people to return for examination at frequent intervals, say three to six months. At each visit premalignant lesions are identified and treated before malignant change takes place. The development of such lesions can be slowed or prevented by avoiding sunlight exposure, by proper selection of clothing, and by constant use of a suitable sunscreen agent.

If actinic keratoses are not treated, many of them will ultimately develop into a squamous cell carcinoma which invades and may metastasize. One textbook [2] states that 20—25 per cent of keratoses become squamous cell carcinomas. Almost all such squamous cell carcinomas arising from actinic exposure are well differentiated, of a low grade malignancy, grow slowly, and metastasize infrequently and late in the course of their progression. This low grade of malignancy and sluggish growth is not characteristic of other forms of squamous cell carcinoma of the skin, particularly those that develop on unexposed areas or on mucous membranes.

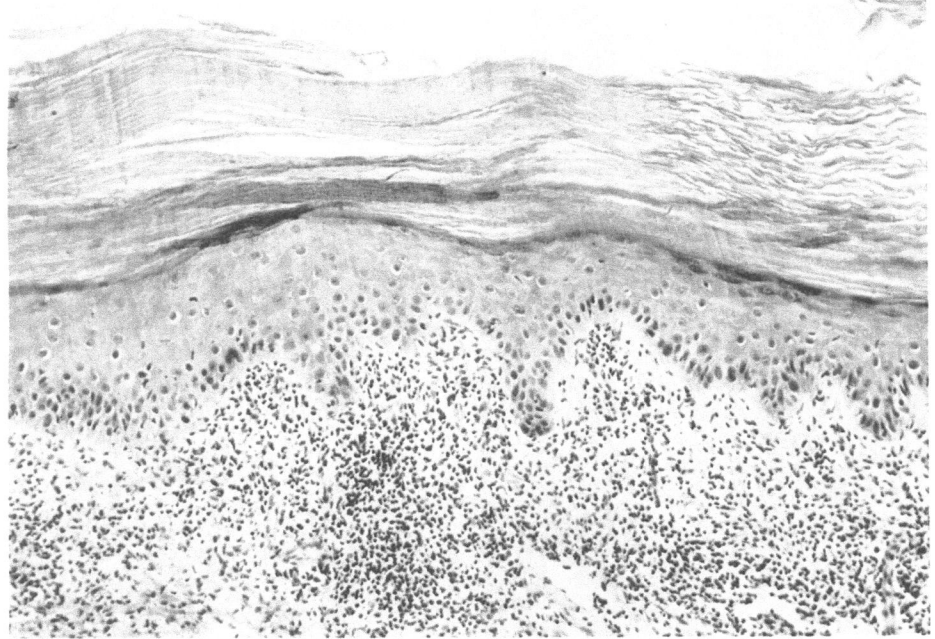

Fig. 3. Hyperkeratosis, dyskeratosis, and a dermal inflammatory response are typical of the early stage of an actinic keratosis

The typical squamous cell carcinoma begins as an actinic keratosis and appears as a slight nodular thickening of the actinic keratosis palpable as a button-like thickening. It slowly enlarges into a distinct, fairly well circumscribed nodule or tumor which may ulcerate. A typical example is shown in Figs. 5, and 6.

Other forms of squamous cell carcinoma follow fairly distinctive patterns that can be recognized by the experienced eye. When a large aggregation of horny material piles up on top of a lesion, a *cutaneous horn* is formed (Fig. 7). Horns are most often actinic keratoses but invasion may have occurred at the base, transforming the tumor into a squamous cell carcinoma. A variety of other lesions, including benign conditions such as warts or seborrheic keratoses, also can produce cutaneous horns.

Bowen's disease represents an intraepithelial squamous malignancy commonly seen on unexposed areas and appearing as an irregularly outlined but sharply

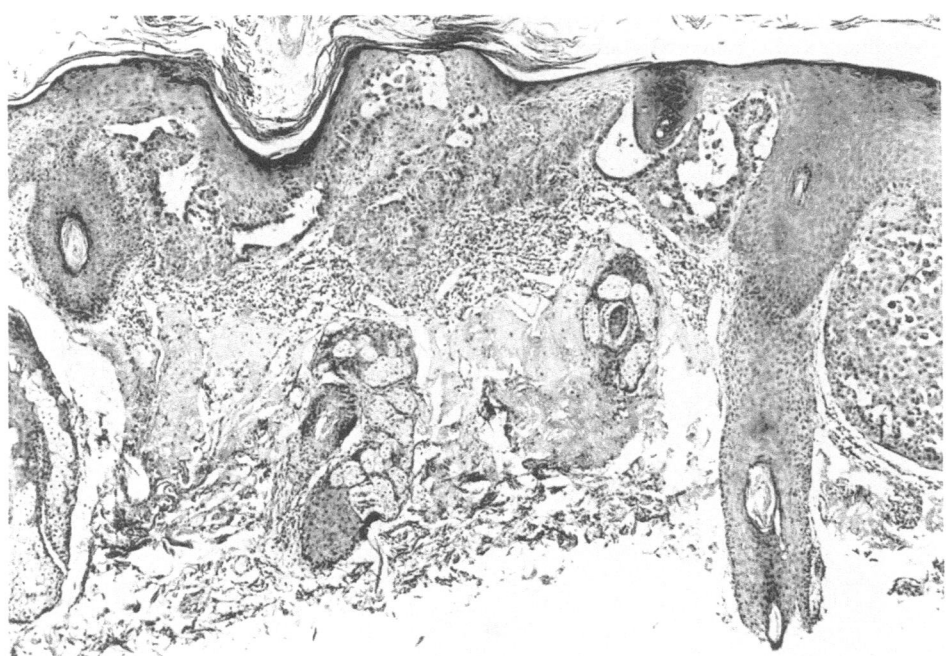

Fig. 4. With progression of actinic keratoses, the premalignant epithelium proliferates downward. Acantholysis is an occasional finding. The collagen degeneration is well shown

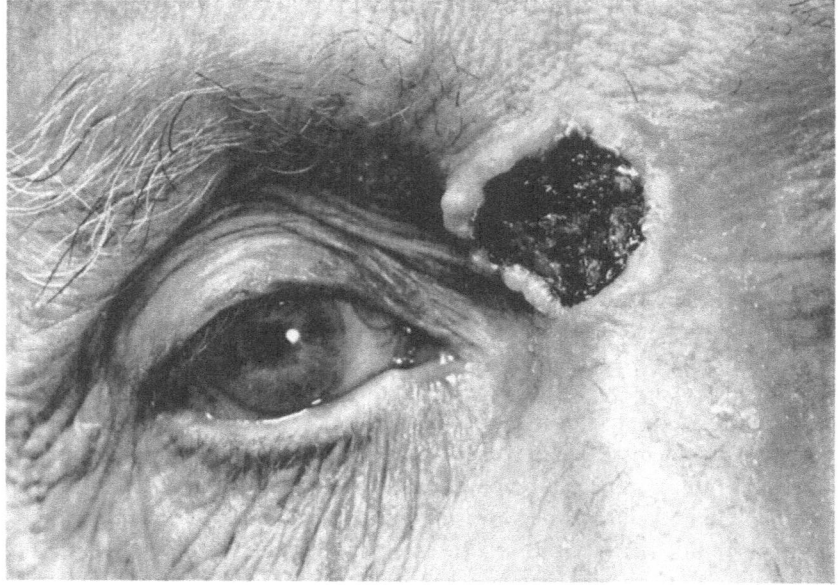

Fig. 5. This is an ulcerating squamous cell carcinoma on an 80 year old man

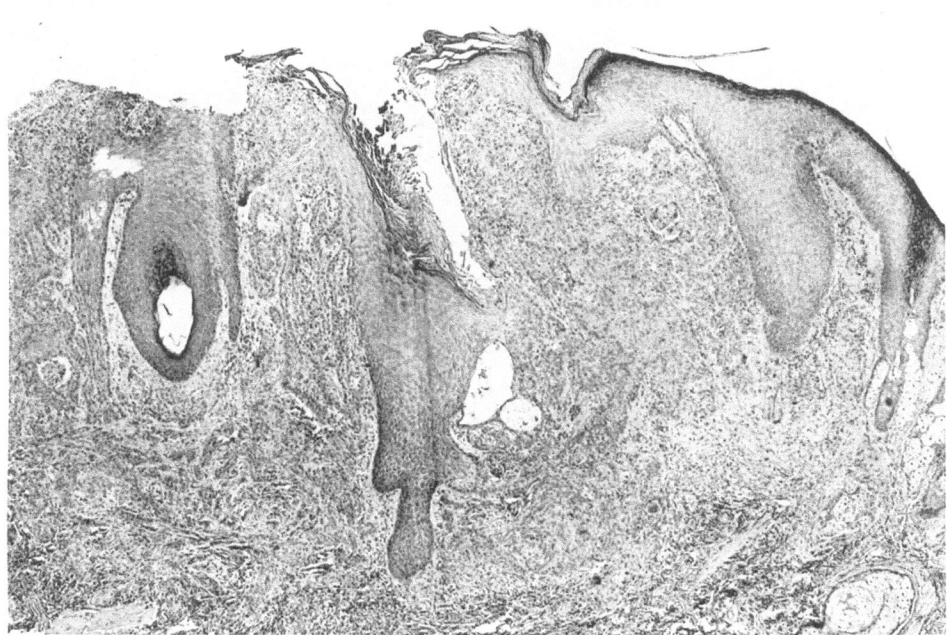

Fig. 6. Invasion of malignant squamous cells can be seen in this ulcerated tumor. The follicular epithelium is not involved in the malignant transformation

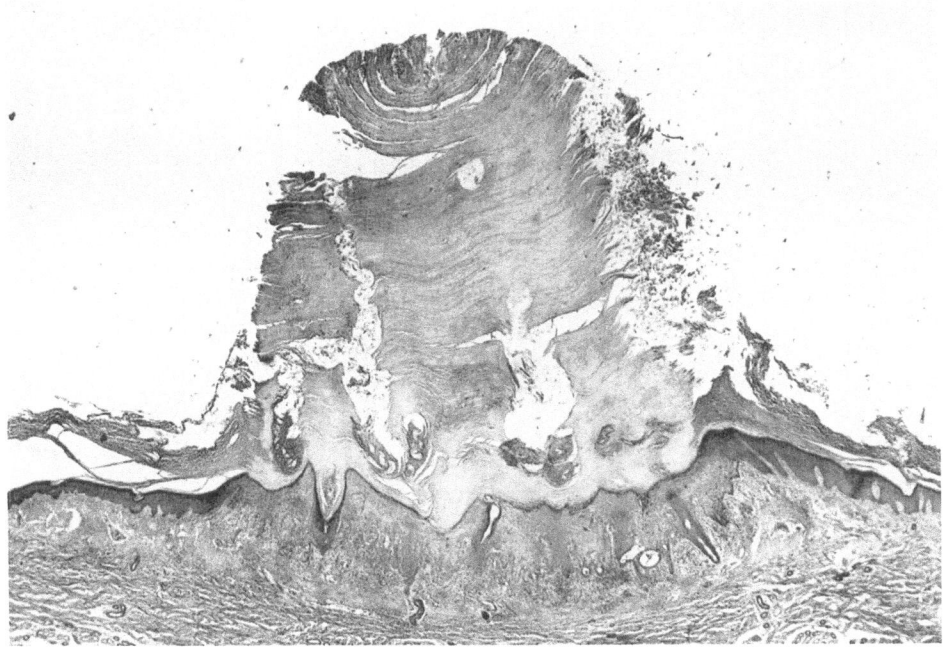

Fig. 7. This cutaneous horn shows the changes of an actinic keratosis at its base

circumscribed erythematous, scaly, papular or macular lesion (Figs. 8, 9). It may be mistaken for an eczematous condition, an actinic keratosis, or a superficial type of

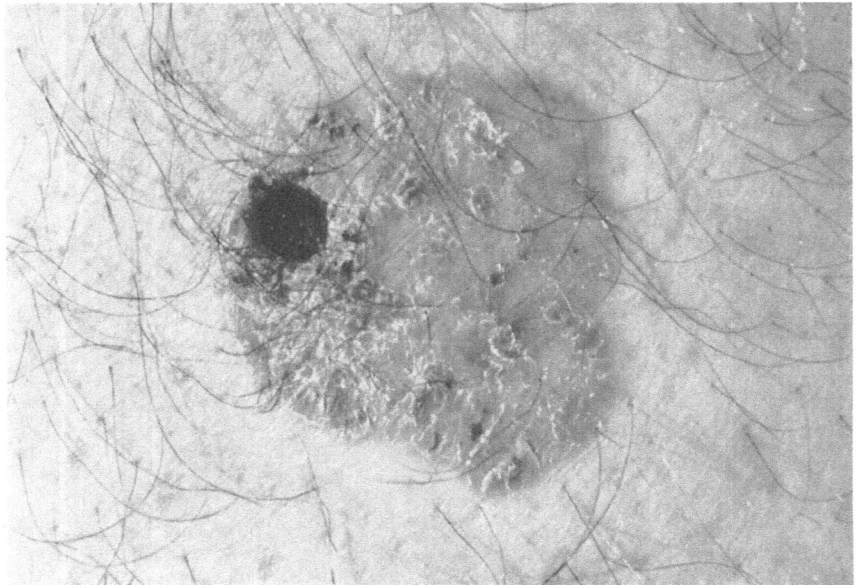

Fig. 8. This scaly patch illustrates Bowen's disease, an intraepidermal squamous cell carcinoma. Compare it with the superficial basal cell epithelioma in Fig. 17. Biopsy may be necessary to distinguish between them

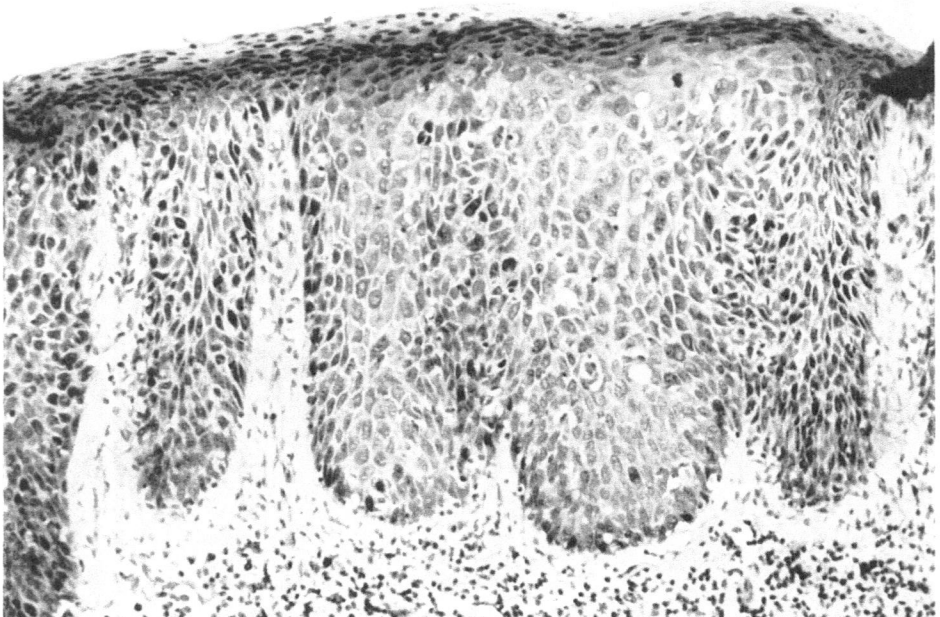

Fig. 9. In Bowen's disease, the entire thickness of epidermis shows dyskeratosis. Invasion may be a late event

basal cell epithelioma, but the correct diagnosis is easily confirmed by biopsy. The association of this type of skin cancer with other forms of internal cancer has been reported [3—5]. In one study a third of patients with Bowen's disease on unexposed skin also had an internal cancer [6]. While it may be important to perform a careful history and physical examination and other indicated tests, we do not feel that an exhaustive or expensive search for an internal malignancy need be done routinely in every patient with Bowen's disease.

Arsenical compounds may cause premalignant keratoses *(arsenical keratoses)* and approximately one-fifth of these eventually become squamous cell carcinomas. These may be widespread and develop without regard to sunlight exposure although classically they are located on the palms and soles. This distribution is unique and strongly indicative of arsenical etiology. Fortunately, much less arsenic is being used medicinally though some commercial and industrial exposure still occurs. We see no reason to use arsenic as a therapeutic agent in any patient. Whether arsenic causes other forms of skin cancer is an unsettled question.

Fortunately squamous cell carcinomas caused by exposure to *ionizing irradiation* are seen less frequently because physicians have become increasingly aware of the danger of radiation exposure. Accidental or iatrogenic exposures still happen, however, and may occasionally precipitate a squamous cell carcinoma. These may be well differentiated but are much more likely to invade aggressively and to metastasize. These cancers frequently have developed on the hands of radiologists and x-ray technicians.

Skin malignancies may arise in *old burn scars*. The classic tumor to do so is a squamous cell carcinoma (Marjolin's ulcer) although basal cell epitheliomas and sarcomas also may localize in such scars.

A unique intraepithelial squamous carcinoma on the male genitalia is known as *erythroplasia of Queyrat*. It is a sharply circumscribed, bright red, velvety, macular or papular plaque. While typically intraepidermal it can invade.

Paget's disease is a unique carcinoma involving the epidermis and appearing as an erythematous and scaly macular patch. It is not a true squamous cell carcinoma but probably represents intraepithelial invasion by an underlying adenocarcinoma of the breast or apocrine gland. It usually occurs on the breast near the nipple. The extra-mammary locations (e.g. axilla, groin, where apocrine glands are numerous) are quite unusual, and an underlying apocrine carcinoma cannot always be found.

Basal Cell Carcinoma

Basal cell epitheliomas are epithelial tumors of the skin probably arising from primitive germ cells and often resembling skin appendages, especially hair follicles. They develop almost exclusively on hair-bearing skin, usually the face, although some have been reported on the thick skin of the palm or sole [7]. They do not develop on mucous membrane. Their incidence is increased by prolonged sunlight exposure.

Basal cell epitheliomas appear at an earlier age than squamous cell carcinomas and may be seen in young adults. In the basal cell nevus syndrome, many skin tumors indistinguishable from basal cell epithelioma appear in childhood and are associated with other cutaneous and skeletal anomalies.

Basal cell epitheliomas extend locally and may be quite destructive. They usually do not metastasize although exceptions to this have been reported [8]. Their growth follows several different patterns and a knowledge of these is essential for accurate diagnosis.

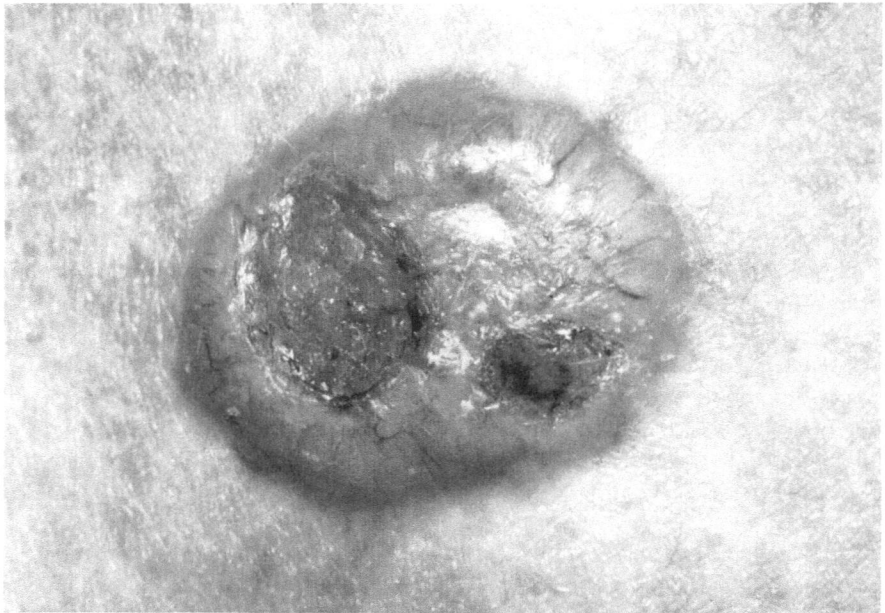

Fig. 10. This is a typical nodulo-ulcerative basal cell epithelioma

The most common type is the *nodulo-ulcerative* type which appears as a small, raised, rounded, pearly or translucent nodule, having small telangiectases on the surface (Figs. 10, 11). The larger lesions ulcerate and if not treated may become locally invasive and destructive. If melanin is in the tumor or the surrounding stroma, the lesions are designated as *pigmented* basal cell epitheliomas. Tumor nodules may undergo cystic degeneration, giving rise to *cystic* basal cell epithelioma (Fig. 12). Irregular growth in narrow strands, sometimes with degenerative cystic change, gives rise to a pattern suggesting gland-like spaces. Such tumors are termed *adenoid* basal cell epitheliomas. These behave in a manner similar to the nodulo-ulcerative type and probably represent minor variations or a slightly different line of differentiation.

The *premalignant fibroepithelioma* (Pinkus) has a unique histologic pattern with interlacing narrow strands of tumor and an overabundance of loose fibrous stroma. It may be raised and firm like a fibroma and is often slightly pedunculated.

Some basal cell epitheliomas develop a sclerotic and atrophic center as they invade and grow peripherally. In these cases a peripheral ring of small pearly nodules typical of the nodulo-ulcerative type surrounds a central atrophic and sclerotic area. This type has been designated *sclerosing* basal cell epithelioma (Figs. 13, 14). This term is sometimes confused with and used interchangeably with the term "morphea-like" basal cell epithelioma but the two types should be separated.

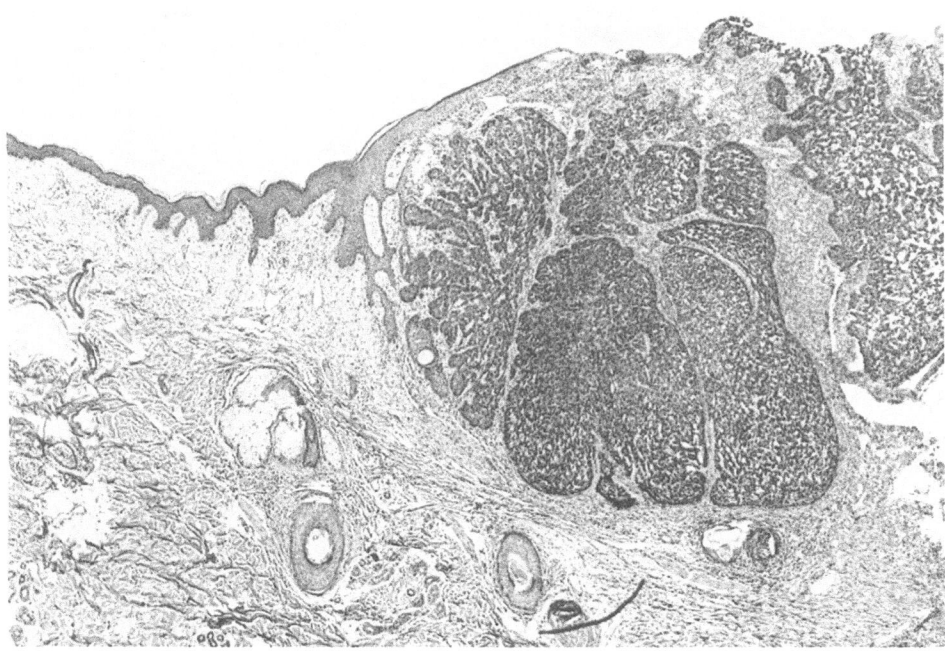

Fig. 11. This is representative of the typical histologic appearance of a nodulo-ulcerative basal cell epithelioma

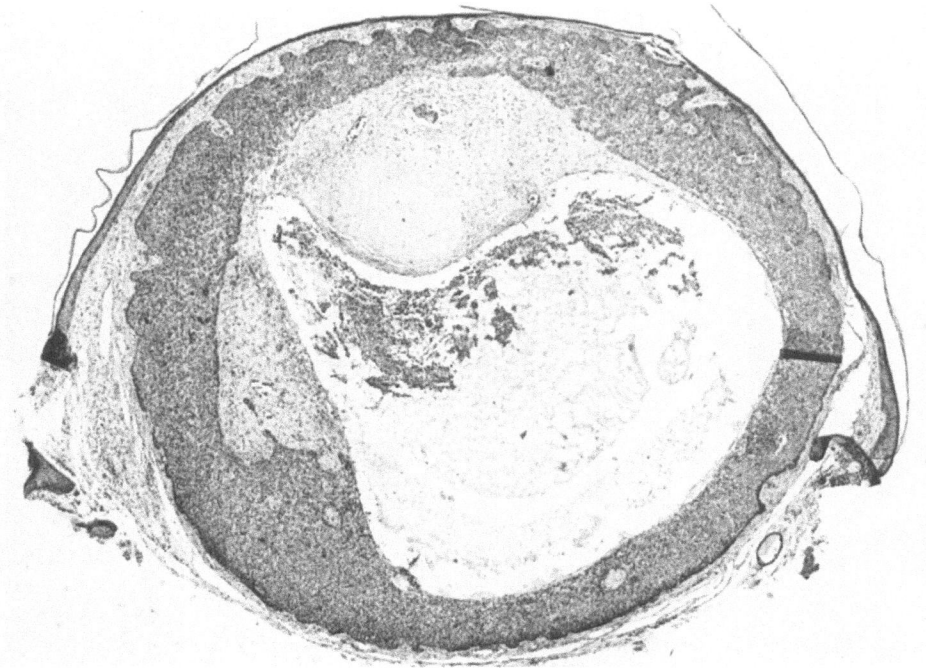

Fig. 12. This is a cystic basal cell epithelioma

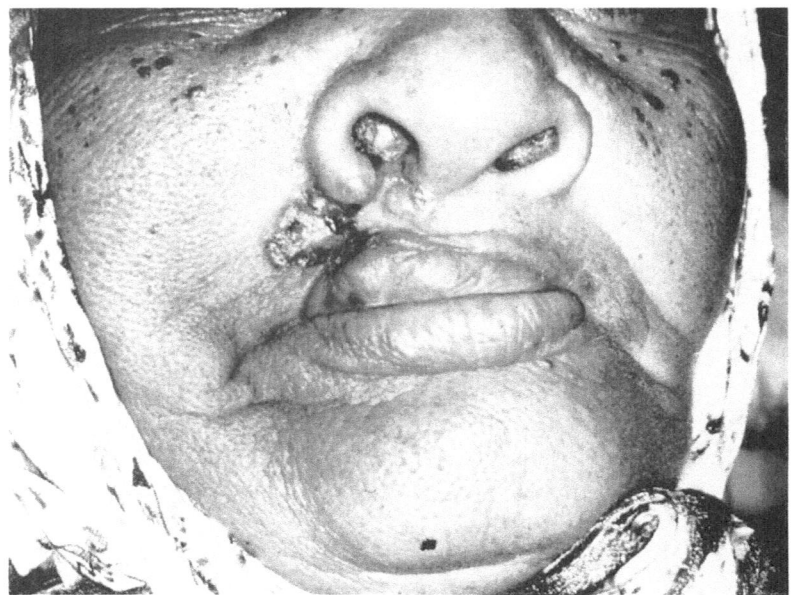

Fig. 13. This basal cell epithelioma on the upper lip of a Negro woman shows central sclerosis with an elevated nodular margin. It should be distinguished from the true "morphea-like" basal cell epithelioma, as shown in Fig. 15

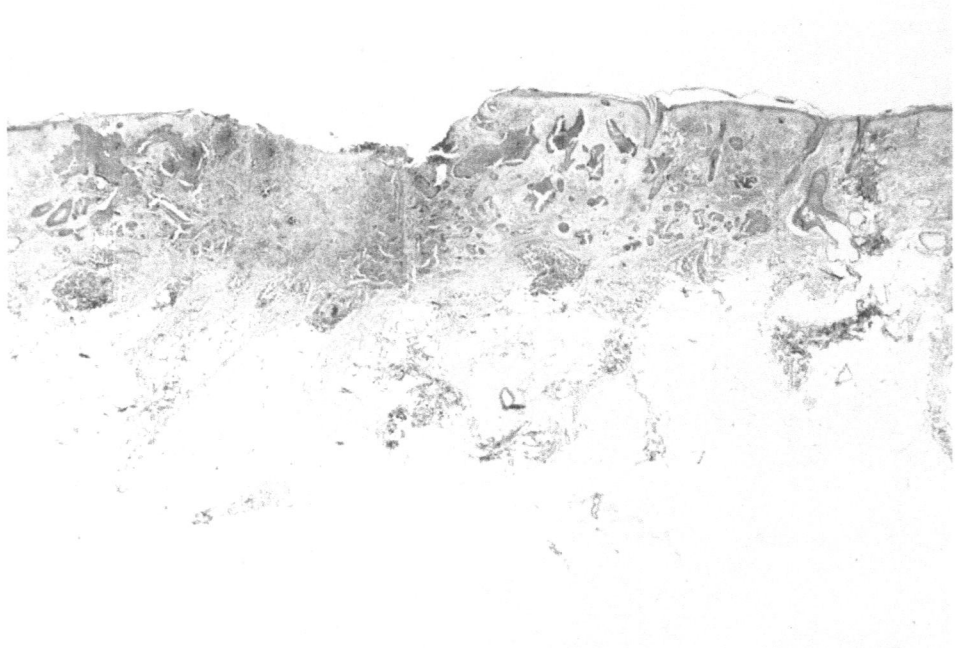

Fig. 14. Sclerosis is seen in the center of this basal cell epithelioma. The tumor extends widely into the dermis, a feature necessitating treatment or removal of a wide margin of normal-appearing skin

The *morphea-like* basal cell epithelioma appears as a slightly depressed, firm, grey-white, irregular area without the peripheral nodules (Figs. 15, 16). It is often mistaken for a scar or localized scleroderma (morphea). It consists of many very small strands of epithelial tumor cells encased in a dense sclerotic stroma. It is particularly prone to recur because it is often not recognized as a skin cancer, the margins are ill-defined and treatment is often inadequate.

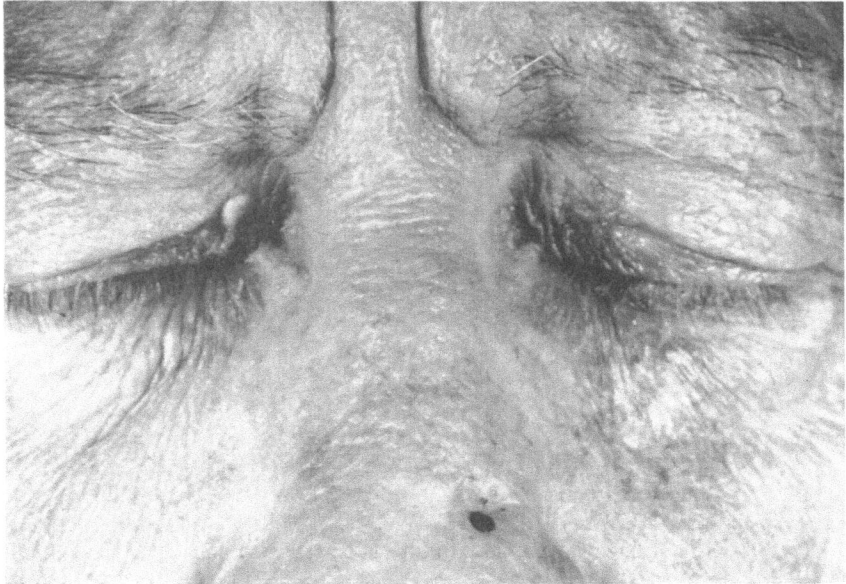

Fig. 15. The small depressed area on the nose (marked by a black dot) is a morphea-like basal cell epithelioma

Some basal cell epitheliomas grow as small nodules scattered along and attached to the basal layer of the epidermis, forming a plaque-like circumscribed lesion without infiltration. They are usually erythematous and scaly, may contain a few small pearly nodules, and may be ulcerated. This type is designated as *superficial* basal cell epithelioma (Figs. 17, 18).

Some skin cancers have features of both basal and squamous cell carcinomas. These have been designated as *basosquamous* or *intermediate cell* types. Virtually all such tumors we have seen could be classified as either basal or squamous cell carcinoma after careful study and histopathologic sectioning of many areas of the tumor. Most such cases we have observed represent squamous metaplasia occurring in basal cell epitheliomas that have ulcerated, recurred or been traumatized or irritated. A few have represented poorly differentiated squamous carcinomas which did not produce keratin or show squamous differentiation but which had many mitotic figures as well as great cellularity and anaplasia. They did not show the typical peripheral palisading, the fibrous stroma, or other features expected in a basal cell epithelioma.

The concept of basosquamous carcinoma should not be confused with "collision" tumor in which a basal cell epithelioma and a squamous cell carcinoma develop in

the same area and grow into each other. This tumor is not uncommon in patients with
severe actinic degeneration of the skin and cancer-proneness.

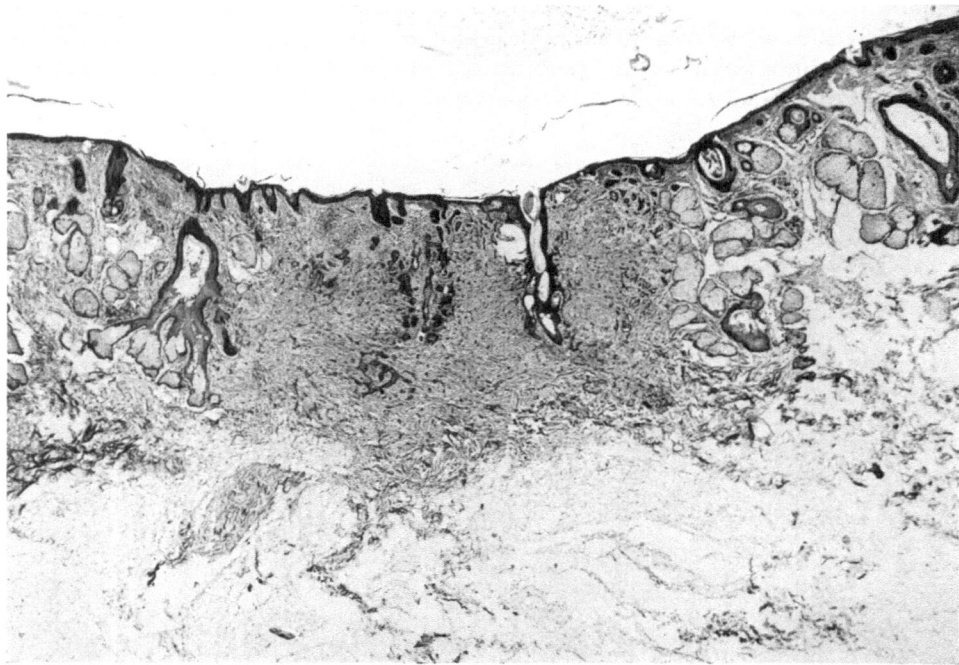

Fig. 16. Small strands of tumor cells encased in dense fibrous tissue represent the typical
findings of a morphea-like basal cell epithelioma

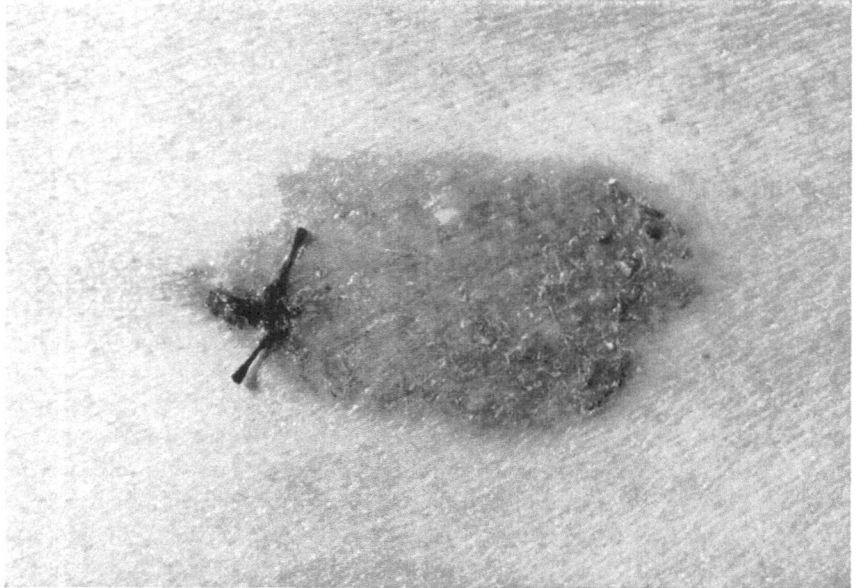

Fig. 17. This flat and scaly superficial basal cell epithelioma had several small translucent
papules in it. Compare with Fig. 8

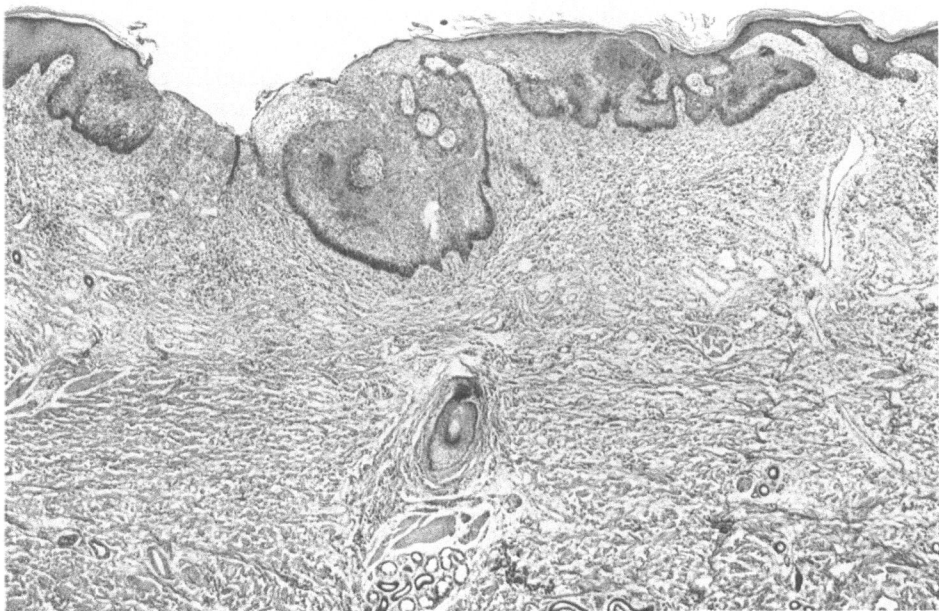

Fig. 18. In this superficial basal cell epithelioma, small tumor nodules are attached to the epidermis

Keratoacanthoma

This benign epithelial skin tumor is unique in that it usually develops rapidly to a size of 1—2 cm. then regresses spontaneously within 6—8 months.

Keratoacanthoma was first described more than 70 years ago by Sir JONATHAN HUTCHINSON under the title "crateriform ulcer of the face". Common synonyms are verrucome, molluscum sebaceum, molluscum pseudocarcinomatosus, primary self-healing squamous epithelioma, and tumor-like keratoses of POTH. Keratoacanthomas are usually solitary but may be multiple and widespread. The multiple type in which there are several or perhaps as many as 100 lesions also has been called self-healing epithelioma of FERGUSON-SMITH. A rare variant with innumerable widely distributed lesions constitutes a third type for which BAER and KOPF suggested the term eruptive keratoacanthoma.

Keratoacanthoma was recognized under a variety of names but was not well accepted in the United States as an entity until about 1954 when the first article appeared under this title in the American literature. Prior to its widespread acceptance most keratoacanthomas were probably called squamous cell carcinoma. In retrospective studies, keratoacanthomas comprised approximately 18 per cent of all squamous type skin tumors. Apparently they developed just as often then but were erroneously diagnosed as squamous cell carcinoma.

Keratoacanthoma has a characteristic clinical appearance as a sharply demarcated papule or nodule with rounded "shoulders" and a central keratin filled crater. They commonly occur on exposed areas, e.g. the face, hands, and forearms. In one series, 17 per cent of keratoacanthomas developed on the face and 19 per cent on the hand or forearm, while the remaining 10 per cent were widely scattered. Sunlight is further implicated as an etiologic factor by the finding that surveys of incidence from different latitudes yield similar ratios of keratoacanthomas to squamous cell carcinomas. Otherwise one would expect that keratoacanthomas would comprise a higher percentage of tumors in northern latitudes, where sunlight-induced cancers are infrequent.

In addition to the usual locations on the face and exposed areas of the hands and forearms, keratoacanthomas have been observed on the eyelid, the pinna of the ear, the mastoid region, the nose, nasal septum, columella, and lip near the vermillion border. Unusual locations have been reported on oral mucous membrane, conjunctiva, larynx and palm of the hand.

Some keratoacanthomas may grow to be quite large, i. e. several centimeters in diameter and may even spread in an annular or irregular configuration.

Some clinically and histologically typical keratoacanthomas have recurred after removal. Many of these recurrences have been successfully removed although a few cases have recurred a second and third time and with each recurrence the growth pattern and the invasiveness and the cytologic irregularity have increased so that a pathologist examining sections from a recurrence will often be unable to distinguish this tumor from a squamous cell carcinoma.

The histopathologic picture of keratoacanthoma usually is as characteristic as the clinical appearance. The crater contains a large irregular mass of keratin or several smaller masses in finger-like recesses. These are surrounded by cohesive masses of acanthotic squamous epithelium made up of cells which contain abundant cytoplasm and relatively small round or oval nuclei showing little atypia. Abnormal keratinization is usually observed in individual cells or as keratin pearls. The basal cell layer usually is intact, although the tumor will extend downward and invasion may be simulated by pseudopods of epithelium. The "shoulders" will be covered by acanthotic epidermis. The dermis will manifest a chronic inflammatory response and, usually, actinic damage to collagen. These features allow the pathologist to make the diagnosis of keratoacanthoma with a reasonable degree of accuracy in the majority of instances, although there are cases in which the typical history or some of the characteristic features are lacking and which cannot be differentiated, with certainty, from squamous cell carcinoma. The pathologist will be aided greatly if he is provided pertinent clinical information such as duration, location, and appearance.

During the period of rapid growth, pathologic changes may be atypical and the lesion cannot always be differentiated with certainty from squamous cell carcinoma. For instance, epithelial proliferation and dyskeratosis are found in both conditions. On the other hand, certain features of keratoacanthomas are rarely seen in squamous cell carcinoma, namely, the crater shaped configuration, cohesiveness of the downgrowing epithelial masses, and retention of a basal cell layer. In addition, the dyskeratosis and atypical cellular changes usually are not as marked in a keratoacanthoma as in a squamous cell carcinoma. During regression, the histologic picture appears progressively more benign and in late stages a keratoacanthoma may resemble an epidermal cyst.

References

[1] FREEMAN, R. G., and J. M. KNOX: Clinical diagnosis of skin tumors by dermatologists. Arch. Dermat. 87, 350 (1963).

[2] ORMSBY, O. S., and H. MONTGOMERY: Diseases of the skin. Philadelphia, Pa.: Lea and Febiger 1954.

[3] GRAHAM, J. H., and E. B. HELWIG: Bowen's disease and its relationship to systemic cancer. Arch. Dermat. 80, 133—159 (1959).

[4] EPSTEIN, E.: Association of Bowen's disease with visceral cancer. Arch. Dermat. 82, 349—351 (1960).

[5] CARPENTER, C. L., V. J. DERBES, and H. W. JOLLY: Carcinoma of the skin—a guidepost to internal malignancy? J. Amer. med. Ass. 186, 621—623 (1963).

[6] PETERKA, E. S., F. W. LYNCH, and R. W. GOLTZ: Association between Bowen's disease and internal cancer. Arch. Dermat. 84, 623—629 (1961).

[7] LEWIS, H. M., C. O. STENSAAS, and M. R. OKUN: Basal cell epithelioma of the sole. Arch. Dermat. 91, 623—624 (1965).

[8] LATTES, R., and R. W. KESSLER: Metastasizing basal cell epithelioma of skin. Cancer 4, 866—878 (1951).

Chapter 3

Treatment

Objectives of Treatment

The primary goal in treating skin cancer is, and always must be, a cure. The patient's motivation for seeking a physician's help is to be rid of a possibly mutilating and life-threatening tumor. Many, perhaps all, patients desire a complete eradication of the tumor without a blemish remaining. However, most patients will accept a scar quite readily when they understand the nature of the tumor.

If the tumor is large and advanced, eradication is virtually the sole objective to be considered in treatment. Fortunately, mainly because of public education programs, regular physical examinations, and wider dissemination of knowledge, both doctors and patients are more aware of skin cancers. Medical aid begins earlier, when the cancers are very small or even when they are merely premalignant conditions.

While cure of the patient must remain the primary objective regardless of the lesion's size, smaller lesions do allow us to consider more seriously such secondary factors as cosmetic results, magnitude of the procedure, pain, time and expense. Treating early lesions also allows a choice of a wider variety of modalities for treatment, each having its own advantages and disadvantages. There is less sense of urgency and the choice of modality can be made calmly and thoroughly.

Furthermore, psychological rehabilitation of patients with skin cancer is important. The physician can help them adapt to the fact that they have had a cancer and perhaps avert cancerophobia. At the same time patients should be informed of the possible dangers so that they will return for follow-up examinations and will protect their skin against further injury.

Because many of today's patients have early lesions and because we understand more about the etiologic factors in skin cancer, physicians are able to concentrate on prophylactic measures. Patients should avoid unnecessary sunlight exposure and protect their skin with clothing and sunscreens during any prolonged sun exposure. Greater encouragement of use of prophylaxis by means of public education programs and individual patient instruction will undoubtedly be very helpful in reducing skin damage and the incidence of skin cancers.

General Principles of the Methods

The methods commonly used for treatment of skin cancer involve excision by surgical technics [1—6] or destruction by use of physical or caustic agents [7—15]. Chemotherapeutic agents now being used experimentally are providing a new and broad field for investigation that allows selective destruction of the tumor cells without sacrifice of the patient's normal skin [15—19]. One such agent, topically applied 5-fluorouracil, is being used successfully to treat premalignant lesions [18, 19]. Chemosurgery and other specialized technics are very useful in certain situations but too time consuming for routine use [20].

Most skin cancers are still treated by one of the three widely known methods—surgical excision, irradiation, or curettage and electrodesiccation. When choosing one of these technics or a more specialized procedure the physician should evaluate individually every cutaneous malignancy. In each instance he should consider the following factors: size, location, depth, distinctness of margins, invasiveness, cell type, and the presence or absence of metastatic nodes. These factors along with the advantages and disadvantages of each modality will usually determine which method is preferable for a particular tumor. Rarely is there a need to combine modalities.

Most skin cancers of the squamous cell or basal cell types can be cured by the skilled use of any of these three technics. When one method has no great advantage over another, the physician should use that method with which he has had the most experience and is most proficient. He must be thoroughly familiar with any technic he chooses to employ. Special training is as much a necessity for use of irradiation or for curettage followed by electrodesiccation as it is for surgical excision.

The cure rate in skin cancer is remarkably high when these three technics are used correctly and could be even higher if patients were taught to seek medical care earlier and if physicians would carefully evaluate and appropriately treat each lesion.

Surgical Excision

Surgical excision of skin tumors is undoubtedly the most widely known and widely used of the three methods. It has the advantage of being a simple direct attack aimed at immediate and complete removal of the cancer. Also it allows the pathologist to examine the tumor carefully to make some prediction about its behavior, to determine its exact nature, and to decide whether removal has been complete.

Most surgical excisions of skin cancer can be performed without an elaborate operating room suite or anesthetic service. The fundamental surgical skills necessary to treat the majority of skin cancers are learned readily. We emphasize, however, that this applies to *most* cases requiring simple surgical excision. Complicated skin

tumors can tax the skill of even the most highly trained cancer surgeons working
with the most modern equipment and technics.

It is very important to include a significant margin of normal skin around *and*
beneath the tumor (Fig. 19). This margin should be 1/2 to 1 cm. at all edges, even
wider in tumors with a diffuse growth at the margins, such as the morphea-type
basal cell epithelioma. Inspecting the surface of the tumor before excision will not
always reveal diffuse growth, deeper growth, or small pseudopods. Thus some normal
skin must be removed to allow for a margin of error.

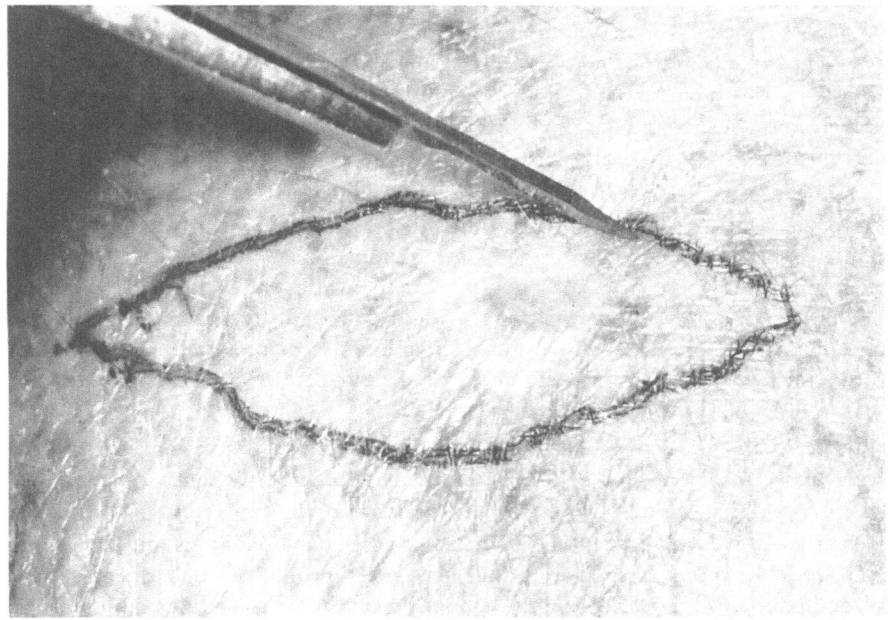

Fig. 19. The line of elliptical excision is marked off for removal of a small nodular basal
cell epithelioma. Larger or unusual types require more radical procedures

Most surgeons in training should concentrate on developing diagnostic skills.
Evaluating the extent of cancer growth is the most critical and important step in
surgical excision because it is at this step where error resulting in failure most often
occurs. There must be careful examination by inspection, palpation and possibly
preliminary biopsy to determine the exact extent of the tumor, both at the margins
and depth. Inconspicuous extensions of tumor can often be detected by the experienced eye and failure avoided. Once this examination is done, and the margins of
the tumor marked off, it is a straightforward matter to apply surgical technic, keeping in mind basic surgical principles found in many standard textbooks, such as
placing suture lines in the lines of cleavage and undermining the wound margins.
Closure of large defects may necessitate skin grafting; thus the surgeon excising large
lesions should be familiar with the principles of that technic.

In his pre-operative evaluation of the extent of the lesion the surgeon should
examine all possible sites of metastasis, particularly the regional lymph nodes. If he
finds an enlarged node in the area of lymphatic drainage of the tumor he may decide

to do a radical lymph node dissection in addition to the excision, or he may choose a different modality than excision.

Surgical excision has the disadvantage that every margin cannot be checked completely and the possibility of recurrence then still remains. When excising skin cancers, surgeons commonly ask a pathologist to examine a frozen section to determine whether wider excision is indicated. The surgeon should keep in mind, however, that the pathologist is handicapped in this situation. Actually he has enough time to check only a few of the margins of a specimen. Even on permanent sections a pathologist cannot always be confident that every margin has been checked since residual tumor could occur at any of 360° around the margin of the specimen. Results of a recent study [21] indicate that marginal extension of tumor may not be a reliable indication that the tumor will recur, since only 35 per cent of basal cell epitheliomas recurred even though marginal extension was observed and re-excision was not carried out.

The surgeon can help the pathologist by indicating at what point he thinks the tumor may be approaching the margin of the specimen. He can place a suture at this point or mark it with ink or dye. The pathologist should not, however, limit his examination to these particular points marked by the surgeon because he may find other less apparent tumor growth on examination of the specimen. The experienced pathologist can often determine more about the extent of tumor and the adequacy of excision if he is able to examine many cut surfaces of the gross specimen rather than a few isolated microscopic frozen sections.

Occasionally older patients with extensive actinic degeneration of the skin will have many focal areas of actinic keratosis, basal cell epithelioma, or squamous cell carcinoma. Because these are often multicentric in origin, microscopic examination of frozen sections will reveal some of these premalignant or malignant changes at the margin of the specimen suggesting that removal is incomplete. In such cases it may be virtually impossible to determine the exact extent of the malignant change, and it may be futile to attempt to remove all the premalignant change. In such cases, the surgeon should concentrate on eradicating the tumors which are likely to be an immediate life threat and rely upon careful follow-up examination and repeated treatment of new lesions as they appear.

Another disadvantage of surgical excision is that all the remaining tissue is viable and has not been treated in a manner to destroy or inhibit the growth of any remaining tumor. Furthermore, wide surgical excision, including normal skin margins, may necessitate removal of vital structures and thus cause deformity or impaired function. If this is not done, one is forced to compromise and remove the tumor inadequately rather than sacrifice a vital structure.

Surgical excision always leaves a scar. This may not be objectionable on the scalp or on covered areas. In fact, the scar may be quite inapparent particularly on the neck or in the eyelid. Elsewhere, however, it may be extremely difficult or vitually impossible to avoid a cosmetically unacceptable scar. This is particularly true on the shoulders and back where constant tension will cause stretching and enlargement of even the most precisely apposed skin margins.

Skin grafting also often leaves an unsightly scar, particularly if the donor site differs in color and texture from the grafted site. A skin graft tends to retain the texture and color of its original site. Every effort should be made to match these features as closely as possible.

Radiation Therapy

When radiation is used to treat skin cancer a variety of technics may be chosen. Those most commonly used utilized superficial x-ray or radium as the source of radiant energy.

Superficial x-ray is used commonly in a total dose of 3,500 to 5,000 r with half value layer of 0.6 to 1.0 mm. of aluminum. Wide variations in technic are practiced by different therapists [7—10]; however, a common schedule is to give 500 r daily for eight to ten treatments for a total dose of 4,000 to 5,000 r. This can be modified to 1,000 r every other day; however, smaller doses over a longer period reduce the likelihood of necrosis and other complications [22]. BELISARIO [15] recommends a peak kilovoltage of 80 to 100 kv, 4 to 6 milliamps, half value layer of half to two mm. of aluminum and a focal skin distance of 15 to 20 cm. He suggests several schedules of fractionation of the total dose. For further details standard references or experts in the field should be consulted.

Radium may be applied either topically or interstitially. The usual dose in 6,000 to 7,000 gamma r. Tables are available for calculating the exact dosage. For external application, radium coated plaques or platinum tubes containing radium can be used.

An excellent technic for interstitial radium implantation utilizes low intensity radium needles [23, 24]. These needles have a 0.5 mm. platinum wall that filters out all alpha and beta irradiation. They contain 1 mg. of radium per running cm. of length and are embedded approximately 1 cm. apart. Needles are left in the tissue for six or seven days, thus delivering 6,000 to 7,000 gamma r (Fig. 20).

A short-time, high-intensity technic may also be advantageous with small cancers [23, 24]. In this technic needles with 10 mg. of radium, an active length of 12 mm., and a 0.3 mm. platinum wall emit both beta and gamma energy. The needles are placed 3—5 mm. apart at the base of the tumor and left in place for $2\frac{1}{2}$ to 3 hours.

Occasionally gamma irradiation is combined with x-irradiation, using a lower dose of each type but a slightly higher total dose (e.g. 4,500 r or x-ray plus 3,000 gamma rays).

When radiation is used to treat skin cancer, the outermost edges of lesions should be carefully defined. A margin of approximately 5 mm. of normal tissue should be included in the treated area. If x-ray is used the adjacent skin is shielded with lead. A special shield should be designed and cut for each lesion.

When considering radiation as a form of therapy the physician should appraise a number of factors—the age of the patient, the location of the tumor, the type of tumor, its extent and the nature of its growth. As a general principle cancericidal radiation therapy should be avoided in young persons because of the long-term sequelae—radiodermatitis, malignancy, and further aggravation of damage to irradiated skin by superimposed sunlight exposure. In elderly patients radiation may be more favorably considered because there is little danger of these late sequelae. Older patients also may be poor risks for surgery.

The location of the tumor should greatly influence the choice of radiation. A cure and good cosmetic result can be expected following irradiation of tumors on the lip, eyelid and nasolabial area. Radiation is less suitable but may occasionally be indicated for cancers on the scalp, neck, ear or anterior chest. However, on the scalp,

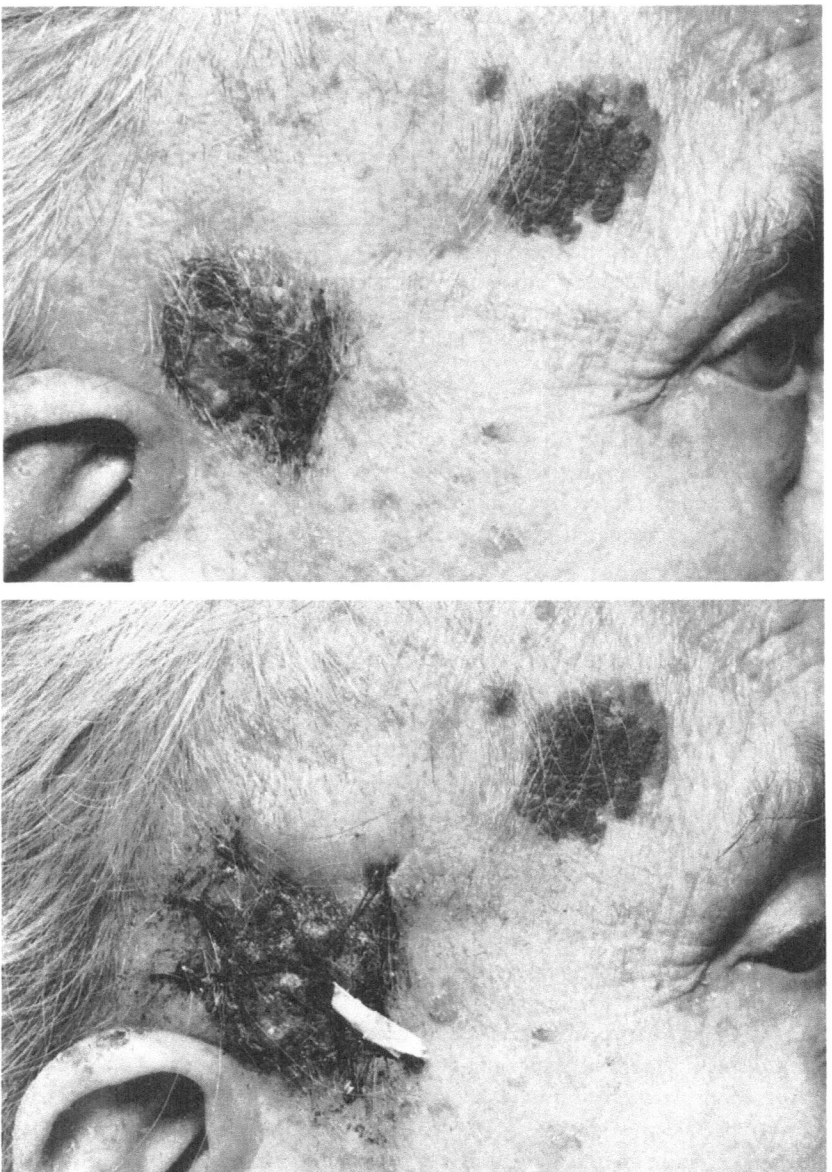

Fig. 20. This shows a basal cell epithelioma before treatment (a) and with the radium needles in place (b). In this patient 5 needles were left in place for 7 days

permanent epilation will result. It rarely should be used on the trunk, extremities, hands or fingers and it should not be used in areas previously treated with x-ray. Many people prefer radiation for treatment of squamous cell carcinomas rather than basal cell epitheliomas. It is often most appropriate for large lesions and surgery or curettage is usually preferable for small lesions. If these fail, radiation can then be used as the second treatment. Radium rather than x-ray is particularly adaptable to lesions of the lip, mouth, tongue or other areas with a curved surface. Radium gives good control of depth of penetration of the rays.

In general, actively growing tumors with mitotic activity will respond favorably. Sclerosing tumors often respond poorly, particularly sclerosing basal cell epitheliomas. These should be excised although in difficult situations radium needle implantations may be used.

Complications of radiotherapy include radiodermatitis, epilation, mucus membrane damage inside the mouth, osteomyelitis (particularly with radiation around bad teeth), chondritis and perichondritis of the ear, nose or nasal septum. Radiation near the eyes may cause cataracts, tear duct occlusion, conjunctivitis or corneal damage.

In our area the use of radiation for skin cancers is decreasing, partly because lesions are seen earlier and are smaller and thus more amenable to other modalities. Secondly, many physicians are turning to curettage and electrodesiccation or to surgical excision as preferable and simpler methods of treatment.

Curettage and Electrodesiccation

The method of curettage followed by electrodesiccation is a combination of surgical removal and use of a physical modality—electrodesiccation. This method is widely used successfully in many parts of the world. In a large series of cases the five-year cure frequencies were as good as those following any other method [11—14]. Curettage and electrodesiccation is particularly useful, indeed the treatment of choice, for routine small basal or squamous cell carcinomas.

Once mastered, this technic is very simple. It can be carried out in the office in one visit; it does not require elaborate equipment; it is inexpensive. It provides a tissue biopsy for pathologic diagnosis and yields excellent cosmetic results.

It has, however, certain disadvantages. It cannot be used in very large infiltrating tumors or in cancers with a tough fibrous stroma such as the morphea-type basal cell epithelioma. It is not appropriate for tumors suspected of being melanomas. These lesions should be excised surgically. While it provides a tissue biopsy, the margins of the specimen are not available for microscopic study. This disadvantage is negated somewhat by the fact that the tissue surrounding the lesion is destroyed by desiccation, thus tumor cells in this area are usually destroyed. Also, during the procedure, if one questions whether the tumor has been completely destroyed a small biopsy can be taken from the site suspected of containing residual tumor and this can be submitted for microscopic examination.

Probably one of the precautions most worthy of emphasis is the importance of learning and following the technic precisely. Failure to do this has led to inadequate treatment and recurrences [25] and this has been the basis for misunderstandings and criticism of the method.

The equipment used and the technical details of the procedure vary from physician to physician. Below is outlined the manner in which we have successfully used the method (Figs. 21—30), in a large series of basal cell and squamous cell carcinomas [12, 14].

1. Local Anesthesia. The tumor (Fig. 22) and the surrounding skin are cleansed.
A topical antiseptic is applied and the area is anesthetized by injection of a local
anesthetic agent such as 1 per cent xylocaine. Alcohol antiseptics may be used. The
alcohol should be allowed to evaporate thoroughly before proceeding, however, since

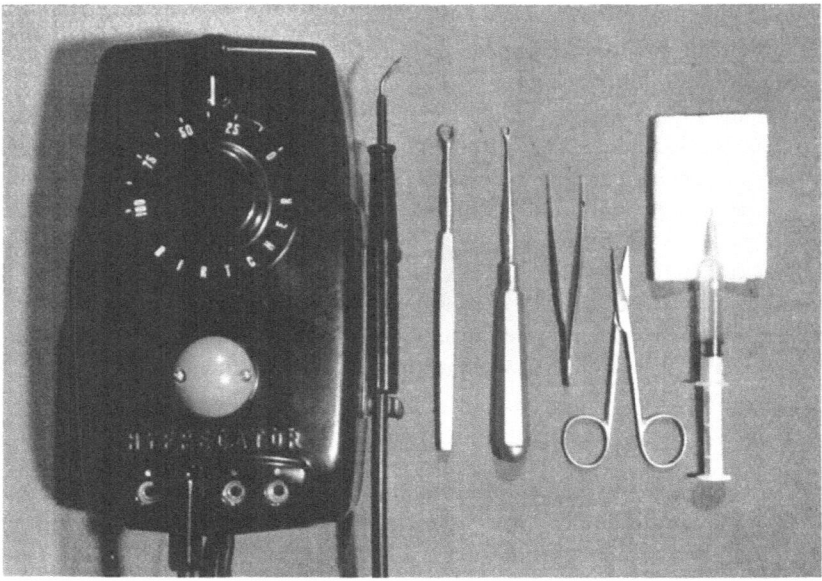

Fig. 21. The equipement used in curettage and electrodesiccation is shown: electrodesiccator,
large curet, small curet, fine rat-tooth forceps, scissors, syringe with local anesthetic

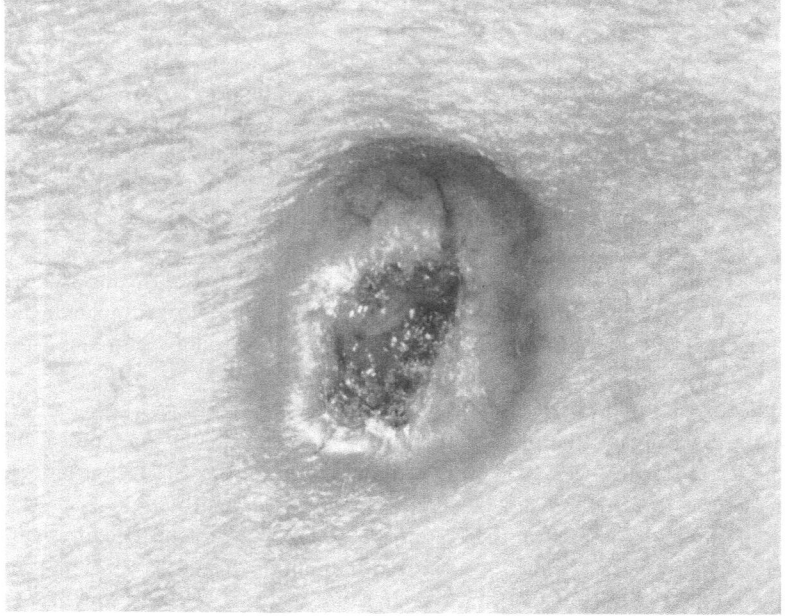

Fig. 22. This represents a typical nodulo-ulcerative basal cell epithelioma before curettage

alcohol is inflammable and may be ignited by the electrodesiccation. Alcohol sponges also should be removed from the area of operation. One per cent xylocaine is usually used because of the immediate anesthesia produced, long duration of action, low allergenicity, and failure to cross-react in procaine-sensitive patients. Any local anaesthetic, however, may be used satisfactorily.

2. Biopsy. After the area is anesthetized, a 6 or 8 mm. curet is used to remove the bulk of the lesion (Fig. 23). We most frequently use the Pfaard or Fry type of curet with a sharp cutting blade, although the Orentreich curet is also popular.

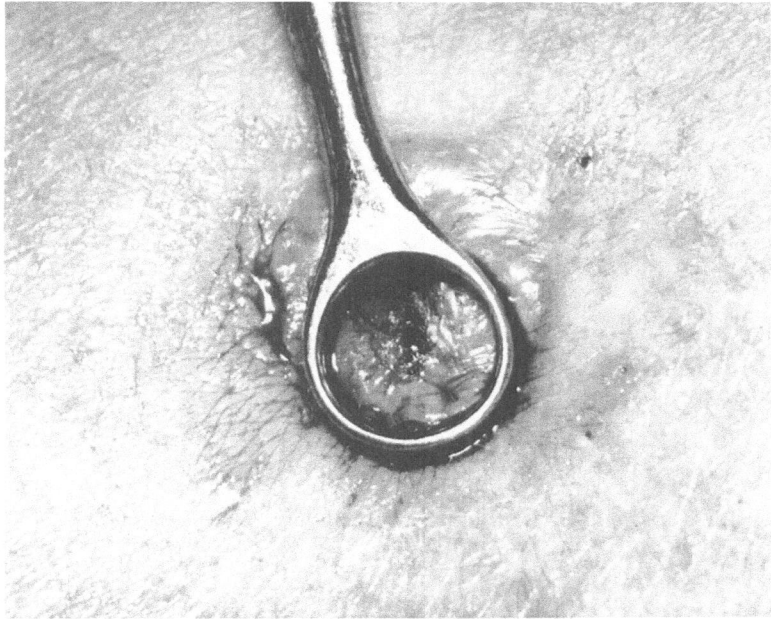

Fig. 23. The large curet is first used to remove the bulk of the tumor for biopsy. The site is then curetted vigorously

Removal is readily accomplished in most skin cancers because of the soft consistency of the tumor. This material is submitted for pathologic diagnosis. It has not been distorted by electrodesiccation and, although it may be fragmented, the tissue is virtually always sufficient for diagnostic purposes. This specimen will often have tumor extending to the margins because it is a biopsy and not an excisional specimen. Since more skin is removed in later stages of the treatment, an evaluation of the adequacy of removal cannot be made from the curetted biopsy.

3. First Curettage. After tissue is obtained for biopsy the remainder of the tumor is curetted vigorously with the 6 or 8 mm. curet until the base of the lesion is reached and all of the soft tumor tissue is removed. Increasing resistance will be encountered as one approaches the normal dermal connective tissue. During this part of the procedure the curet can be used to determine the extent of the tumor and to delineate margins and subsurface irregularities. Various tumors have their own characteristic feel when curetted which skilled operators learn to recognize. After this initial curettage many operators use a smaller curet such as the small cup-shaped or open-end chalazion curet. With this smaller instrument, otherwise inapparent pseudopods and subsurface irregularities can be explored and removed.

   4. First Electrodesiccation. After curettage, electrodesiccation is used to destroy any abnormal cells remaining at the base or sides of the operative site and to provide hemostasis (Fig. 24). Pressure hemostasis may be required temporarily during the

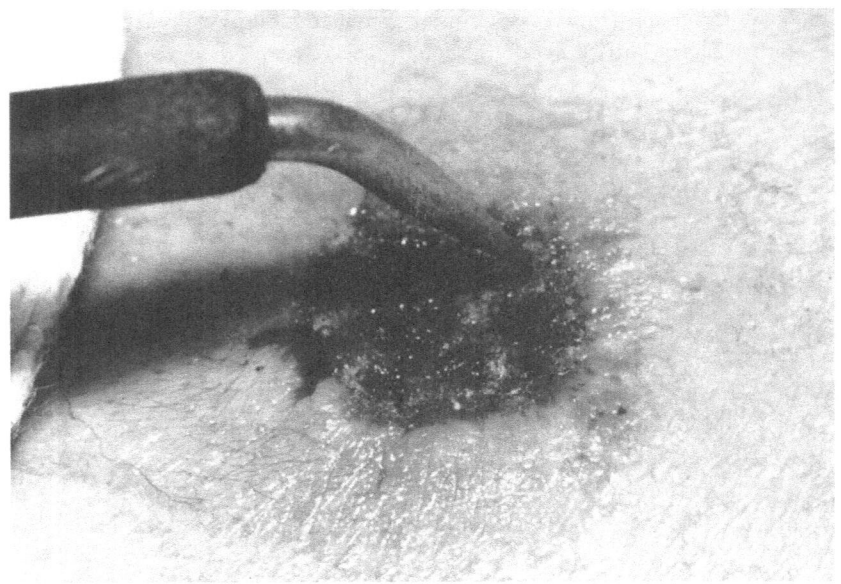

Fig. 24. Electrodesiccation is used to destroy additional tissue and to provide hemostasis

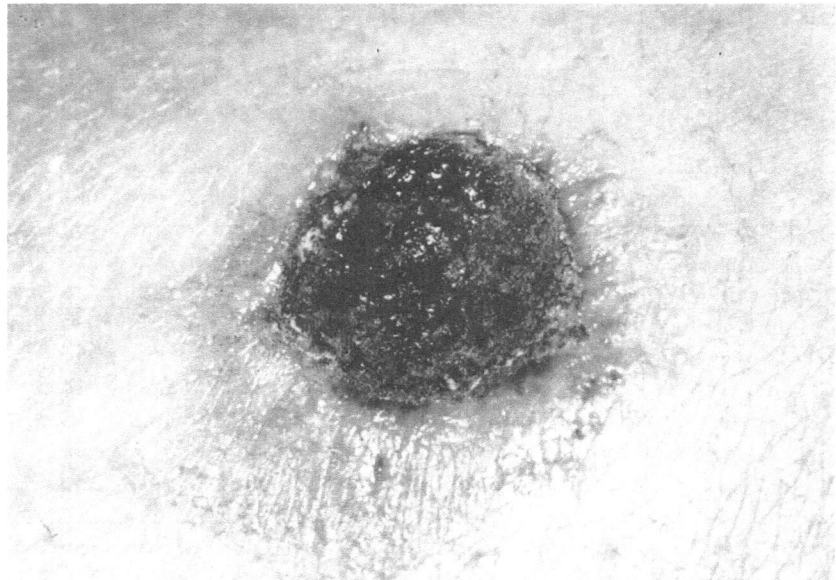

Fig. 25. This is the dry shrunken appearance after the first electrodesiccation

initial stages of electrodesiccation. Electrodesiccation is carried out using a single needle point electrode connected to a single high voltage (Oudin) terminal of a spark-gap apparatus. The needle electrode is held in contact with, or at a slight sparking distance from, the area to be treated. The current employed is one of comparatively high voltage and low amperage with the oscillations damped. Bipolar electrodesiccators in a variety of instruments are available and are equally satisfactory. We use a simple small spark-gap diathermy hyfrecator (Birtcher Corporation, Los Angeles, Calif.) with a frequency of 2,500,000 oscillations per second. It operates on a 50—60 cycle AC current at 110 volts.

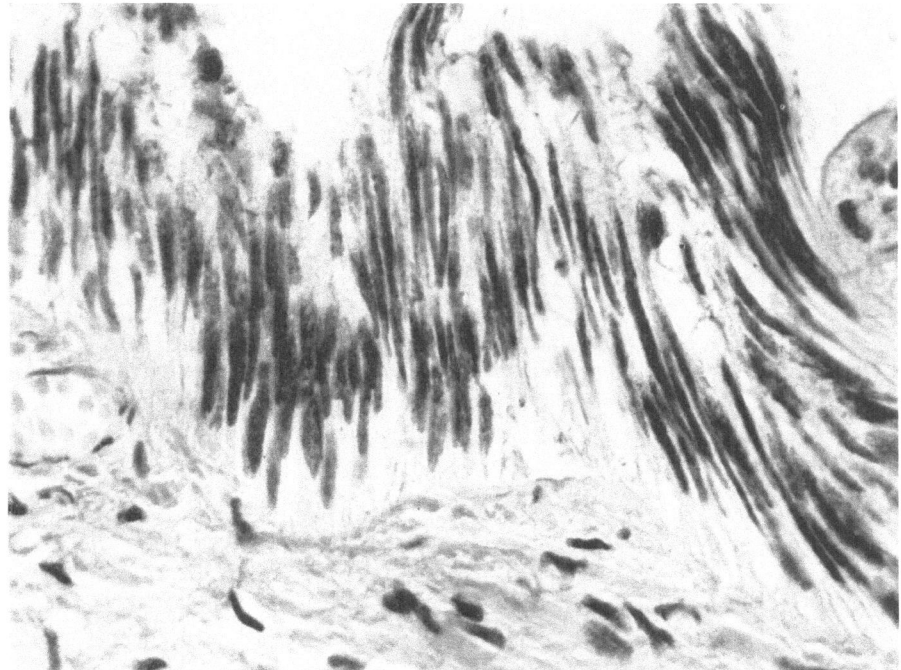

Fig. 26. Electrodesiccation distorts the nuclei and destroys cell outline. [Reprinted with permission of Arch. Dermat. **82**, 197—204 (1960).]

A dry shrunken appearance of the treated area signifies sufficient treatment (Fig. 25). The whole surface mass assumes a mummified appearance and the cells in this area are shrunken with distorted and elongated nuclei (Figs. 26, 27, 28). Hemostasis is provided with this technic by the coagulating effect on the smaller blood vessels. The amount of tissue destroyed by electrodesiccation depends directly on the intensity and duration of the desiccation. The operator therefore can control to a great extent the amount of tissue destroyed and can extend the margins of treated tissue well beyond the original curettage site.

5. Second Curettage. A second curettage is then performed removing the charred and non-viable tissue produced by the electrodesiccation (Fig. 28), and any additional soft readily removable tissue. Normal skin resists curettage.

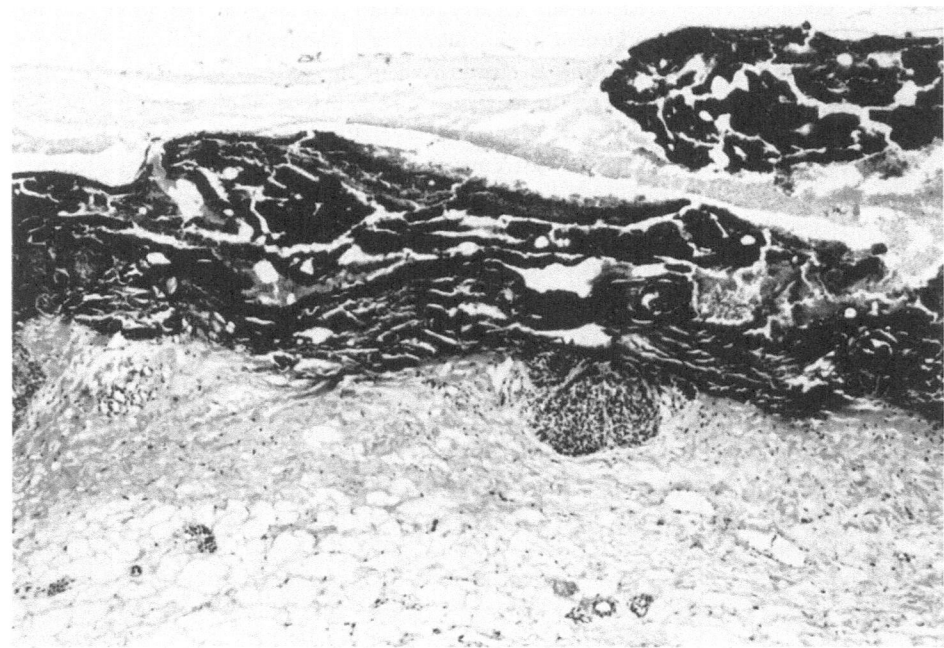

Fig. 27. Electrodesiccation alone, as shown here, would have resulted in a recurrence. [Reprinted with permission of Arch. Dermat. **82**, 197—204 (1960).]

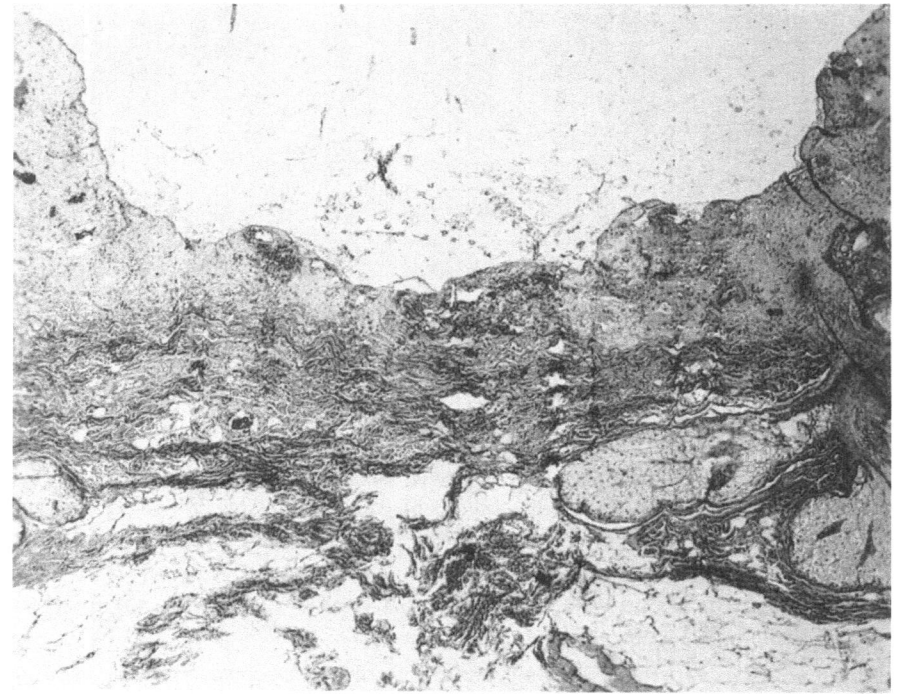

Fig. 28. Curettage alone also would have resulted in a recurrence. [Reprinted with permission of Arch. Dermat. **82**, 197—204 (1960).]

6. Second Electrodesiccation. Electrodesiccation is repeated, extending the desiccated border 2 to 4 mm. beyond the curetted border and achieving hemostasis (Fig. 30).

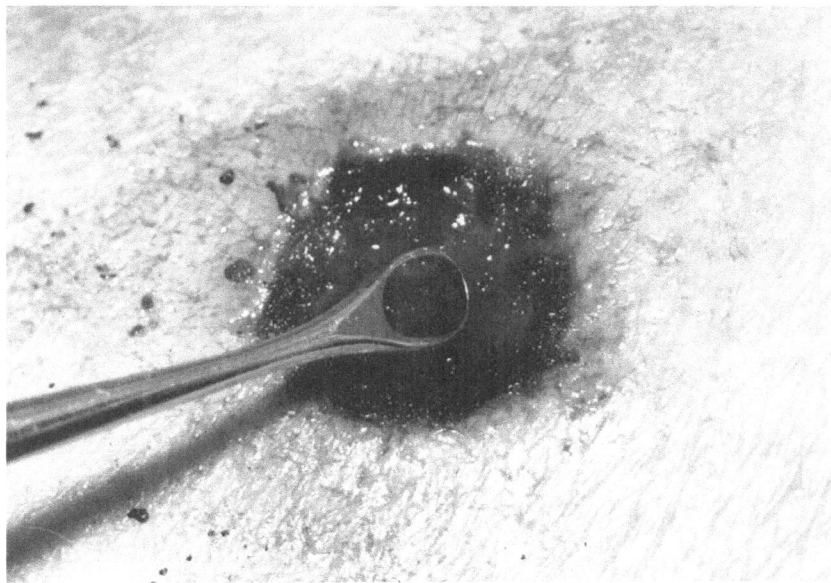

Fig. 29. The charred coagulum is then curetted away

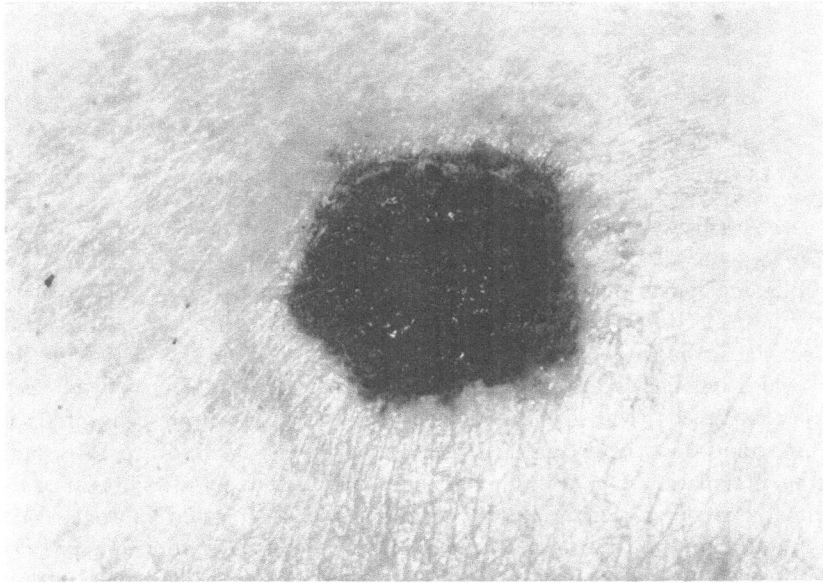

Fig. 30. Electrodesiccation is repeated leaving a dry shrunken wound as shown here

7. Wound Care. A thin charred coagulum remains on the surface and this wound is left open. A local antiseptic agent (for example, rubbing alcohol) may be applied

once or twice daily. Re-epithelialization of the wound takes place from its margins
and from appendages in its base. The crust remains dry for two or three days and
then a mild exudation may occur. After seven to ten days the crust sloughs leaving
a moist surface which soon becomes re-epithelialized. Since electrodesiccation destroys
any bacteria and the wound is protected by an eschar and by antiseptic, secondary
infection is rare. It happens most often when the wound is not left open and an
antiseptic agent is not applied.

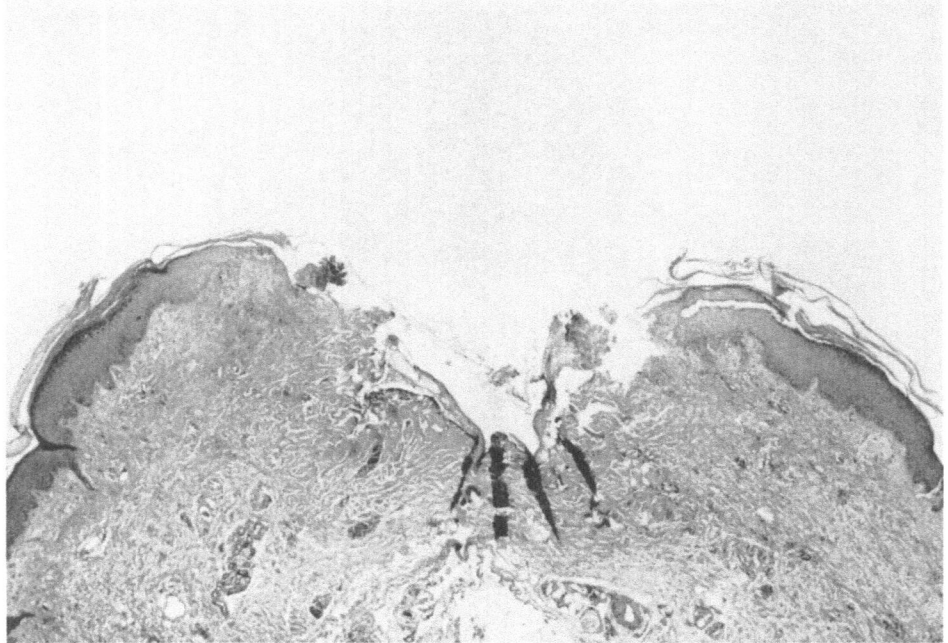

Fig. 31. This shows the treatment site one week following curettage and electrodesiccation
of a squamous cell carcinoma (11 mm. diameter). Serial sections revealed no neoplastic cells.
[Reprinted with permission of Arch. Dermat. 82, 197—204 (1960).]

Cells undergoing mitosis, as with irradiation, are more vulnerable to destruction
by the heat of electrodesiccation than are adjacent normal cells. For a short distance
beyond the actual spark, malignant cells are destroyed by heat. The dry, sterile, open
field which is left after electrodesiccation is a poor site for regrowth of misplaced,
viable cancer cells. This is an advantage over excision since suturing of the wound
margins could trap viable cells. The post-treatment slough, which separates and leaves
healthy granulation tissue, yields an additional margin of safety. Scars following
curettage and electrodesiccation tend to diminish gradually and improve remarkably
in appearance, in contrast to the cutaneous changes after irradiation (Figs. 31, 32).

Most patients are seen again in six weeks. At this time the wounds are usually
well healed, the eschar has dropped off, and re-epithelialization is complete.

Curettage and electrodesiccation should not be used when lesions are unusually
large, ill-defined, invasive, destructive, or when they extend into underlying tissues
such as fascia, cartilage or bone. Excision is the only satisfactory treatment when the

tumor is a fibrotic or sclerotic one such as the morphea-type basal cell. Curettage and electrodesiccation also should not be used on mucous membranes such as the lips and penis.

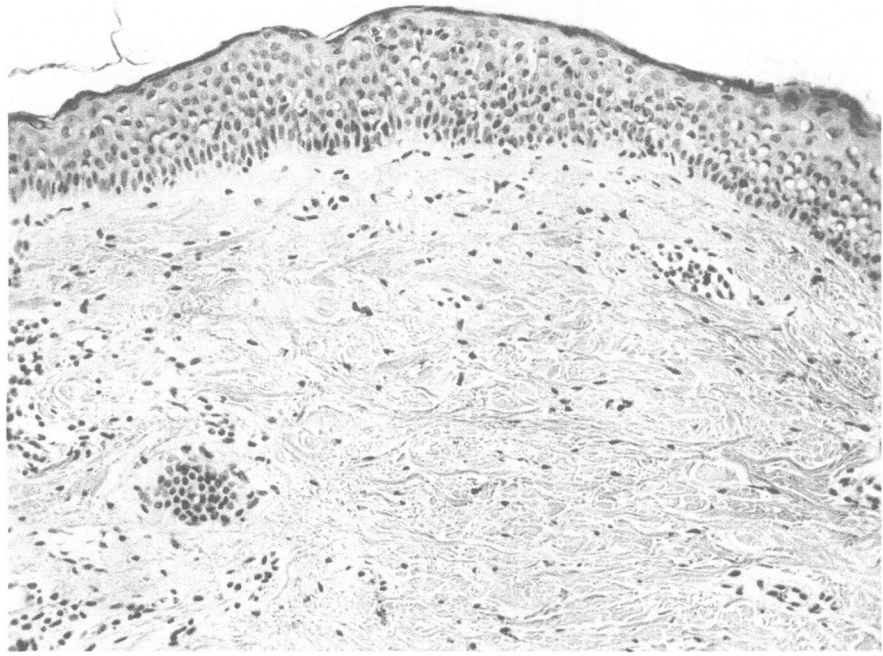

Fig. 32. One year after curettage and electrodesiccation of a basal cell epithelioma on the forehead the site was excised and is shown here. The epidermis and dermis seem relatively normal, although collagen bundles are hypertrophic and appendages are absent. [Reprinted with permission of Arch. Dermat. **82**, 197—204 (1960).]

Chemosurgery

Chemosurgery is a widely known and accepted technic, the principles and methods of which have been set down by Dr. Mohs [20]. Chemosurgery is valuable in certain persistent tumors and avoids unnecessary destruction of tissue in order to remove the tumor completely. It is technically difficult and time consuming and a great deal of experience and patience is required to obtain full sized sections and to map out the lesion carefully in order to locate residual tumors [26]. Tromovitch et al. [27] have used the Mohs technic combined with curettage and electrodesiccation as a double check on areas of the curetted wound where possible persistence of tumor is suspected.

Chemotherapy

Recent widespread interest in using chemotherapeutic agents to treat internal cancers has stimulated investigation of some of these agents for use with skin cancer. Some cytotoxic agents have been in use for a long time. Belisario [15, 28, 29] has used podophyllin and vitamin K preparations for many years and recently reported on the use of colchicine derivatives, demecolcine, N-desacetyl, thiocolchicine, methotrexate and triaziquone (2,3,5-trisethylene-imino-(1,4)-benzoquinone). He achieved favorable results with selective destruction of basal cell epitheliomas, actinic keratoses, Bowen's disease and keratoacanthomas although the agents were ineffective against squamous cell carcinomas. Triaziquone (Trenimon), 5-fluorouracil, 5-mercaptouracil, methotrexate and other similar agents have also been tested [17, 30].

DILLAHA and associates should receive the credit for establishing the clinical usefulness of the cytotoxic agent 5-fluorouracil in the treatment of premalignant actinic keratoses. In 1963 they reported the selective effect of a 20 per cent concentration of 5-fluorouracil in a hydrophilic ointment. This was applied to the skin of the face and neck twice daily for four weeks [18]. More recently [19] they have demonstrated that 5 per cent 5-fluorouracil ointment applied twice daily was as effective as 20 per cent. One per cent in propylene glycol is also effective. Their studies also indicate that the systemic absorption is approximately 6 per cent, well below the toxic level. While they had some success with this agent in treating squamous and basal cell carcinomas, the response was inconsistent. Some actinic keratoses of the hands and arms did not respond completely.

Our results using 5-fluorouracil confirm the effectiveness of this relatively simple method of treating actinic keratoses. The ointment should not be applied near the lid or mucocutaneous junctions. In some patients phototoxicity may develop and the ointment should not be used when prolonged sunlight exposure cannot be avoided.

Malignant Melanoma

Recent improvements in the treatment of malignant melanoma still do not approach the success gained in treating other forms of skin malignancy. Among many possible reasons for this difference, the major ones appear to be: 1) a difference in biologic behavior including a greater tendency to metastasize; 2) delay in recognition due to resemblence to benign lesions and wide variation in the clinical appearance, and 3) scanty knowledge of the etiology and epidemiology. Until a new miracle treatment is discovered, the greatest hope appears to lie in increasing public awareness of the early signs of malignant melanoma and training the physician for proper diagnosis and prompt appropriate treatment.

In management of tumors that are possibly malignant melanomas, accurate diagnosis is paramount. In fact it is absolutely essential for planning the proper treatment. A study of the diagnostic accuracy of a group of trained and experienced dermatologists indicates that they were able to recognize malignant melanomas correctly in approximately 66 per cent of the cases [31], whereas in other studies the diagnostic accuracy of a large group of physicians was only about 40 to 45 per cent. Even trained dermatologists had greater difficulty recognizing malignant melanomas than other forms of skin malignancy. For example, the diagnostic accuracy for carcinomas approached 90 per cent [31]. While there has been some recent improvement in diagnostic accuracy there almost certainly has been an increase in the number of patients who present themselves in a very early stage for diagnosis. This increases the importance as well as the difficulty in diagnosis.

Lesions suspected of being malignant melanoma should not be curetted, desiccated, or treated with chemotherapeutic agents in any way that would distort the mor-

phology of the tumor and interfere with accurate histologic diagnosis. An excision
biopsy will allow accurate pathologic diagnosis of a small lesion, which needs no
further treatment if it is benign. If it is malignant further consideration of treatment
will depend on its size, its location, the degree of malignancy, and the presence or
absence of metastases.

A variety of methods of treatment for malignant melanoma has been used, including surgery, radiotherapy and chemotherapy. In the United States, surgery is
by far the most common method, while in recent years chemotherapy has been used
in the form of perfusion with phenylalamine mustard and other chemotherapeutic
agents [32—34]. Elsewhere radiotherapy has been used successfully in spite of the fact
that this tumor is relatively radio-resistant and requires very high dosages.

For an early, small, or superficial melanoma, the recommended treatment is
usually wide local excision removing a margin of 2 to 4 cm. of normal skin and
removing subcutaneous tissue down to fascial planes. More advanced cases are
evaluated in consultation with a surgeon and pathologist to determine whether regional or en bloc dissections should be carried out or whether perfusion therapy with
phenylalamine mustards is desirable.

None of the modalities of treatment presently available is entirely satisfactory.
Each has its own advantages, disadvantages and contraindications which require
consideration for each individual case. When the modality of treatment is carefully
selected, the results of radical surgery and the results of perfusion sometimes combined with local surgery appear to be approximately equal in terms of long-term
survival. Further experience with perfusion techniques and availability of newer,
more effective anti-tumor chemotherapeutic agents may yield better results in the
future.

References

[1] WARD, G. E., and J. W. HENDRICK: Malignant epithelial tumors of the skin of head and
    neck. Amer. J. Surg. 79, 771 (1950).
[2] RANK, B. K., and A. R. WAKEFIELD: Surgery of basal cell epitheliomas. Brit. J. Surg.
    45, 531—547 (1957—1958).
[3] MACOMBER, W. B., M. K. H. WANG, and J. G. SULLIVAN: Cutaneous epithelioma: a study
    of 853 lesions. Plast. reconstr. Surg. 24, 545—562 (1959).
[4] BATTLE, R. J. V., and T. J. S. PATTERSON: Surgical treatment of basal cell epithelioma.
    Brit. J. Plast. Surg. 13, 118 (1960).
[5] HAYES, H.: Basal cell carcinoma: the East Grinstead experience. Plast. reconstr. Surg.
    30, 273—280 (1962).
[6] McKEE, D. M.: Treatment of basal cell carcinoma. Sth. med. J. (Bgham, Ala.) 57,
    209—215 (1964).
[7] MAGNUSSON, A. H. W.: Skin cancer: A clinic study with special reference to radium
    treatment. Acta Radiologica, Supp. XXII, Stockholm, pp. 1—287, 1935.
[8] PATERSON, R., M. TOD, and M. RUSSELL: The results of radium and X-ray therapy in
    malignant disease. Second Statistical Report from the Holt Radium Inst.,
    Manchester, Edinburgh: E. & S. Livingstone, Ltd. 1946.
[9] EBERHARD, T. P.: Treatment of epitheliomas of the skin. Radiology 49, 620—627
    (1947).
[10] WOOLDRIDGE, W. E., and E. LORENC: Skin cancer treated with combined superficial
     X-rays and gamma radium rays. Mod. Med. 62, 743—750 (1965).
[11] FERRARA, R. J.: The private dermatologist and skin cancer: Clinic study of 226 epi-
     theliomas derived from five dermatologic practices. Arch. Dermat. 81, 225—234
     (1960).

[12] KNOX, J. M., T. W. LYLES, E. M. SHAPIRO, and R. D. MARTIN: Curettage and electro-desiccation in treatment of skin cancer. Arch. Dermat. 82, 197—204 (1960).

[13] SWEET, R. D.: The treatment of basal cell carcinoma by curettage. Brit. J. Dermat. 75, 137—158 (1963).

[14] FREEMAN, R. G., J. M. KNOX, and C. L. HEATON: Treatment of skin cancer. Cancer 17 535—538 (1964).

[15] BELISARIO, J. C.: Cancer of the skin. London: Butterworth & Co., Ltd. 1959.

[15 a] BAER, R. L., and A. W. KOPF: Complications of therapy of basal cell carcinomas. Year Book of Dermatology, 1964—1965. Year Book Medical Publishers, Inc., pp. 7—26.

[16] VAN SCOTT, E. J., R. K. SHAW, R. G. CROUNSE, and P. T. CONDIT: Effects of methotrexate on basal cell carcinomas. Arch. Dermat. 82, 762—771 (1960).

[17] HELM, F., E. KLEIN, H. L. TRAENKLE, and E. P. RIVERA: Studies on the local administra-tion of 2,3,5-triethylene-imino-1,4-benzoquinone (Trenimon) to epitheliomas. J. invest. Dermat. 45, 152—159 (1965).

[18] DILLAHA, C. J., G. T. JANSEN, W. M. HONEYCUTT, and A. C. BRADFORD: Selective cyto-toxic effect of topical 5-fluorouracil. Arch. Dermat. 88, 247—256 (1963).

[19] — — —, and G. A. HOLT: Further studies with topical 5-fluorouracil. Arch. Dermat. 92, 410—417 (1965).

[20] MOHS, F.: Chemosurgery in cancer, gangrene and infections. Springfield, Ill.: Charles C. Thomas 1956.

[21] GOODING, C. A., G. WHITE, and M. YATSUHASHI: Significance of marginal extension in excised basal-cell carcinoma. New Engl. J. Med. 273, 923—924 (1965).

[22] TRAENKLE, H. L., and D. MULAY: Further observations on late radiation necrosis fol-lowing therapy of skin cancer: Results of fractionation of total dose. Arch. Dermat. 81, 908—913 (1960).

[23] LEHMAN, C. F., and J. L. PIPKIN: Radium in malignant cutaneous disease. J. Amer. med. Ass. 154, 4—8 (1954).

[24] WANSKER, B. A.: X-Ray and radium in dermatology. Springfield, Ill.: Charles C. Thomas 1959.

[25] ACKERMAN, L. V., and J. A. DEL REGATO: Cancer, 3rd ed. St. Louis: C. V. Mosby Co., 1962, p. 193.

[26] FORUM: Is chemosurgery advisable for superficial skin cancers of the face. Mod. Med., Oct. 1 (1962).

[27] TROMOVITCH, T. A., G. A. BEIRNE, C. G. BEIRNE, and R. W. LEEPER: Cancer chemosurgery (Mohs technic). Arch. Dermat. 92, 291—292 (1965).

[28] BELISARIO, J. C.: Chemotherapy of skin cancer, rodent and squamous carcinomas and Bowen's disease. Proc. XII Int. 1. Congr. Derm., Washington, D. C., Sept., 1962, pp. 341—350.

[29] — Topical cytotoxic therapy for cutaneous cancer and precancer. Arch. Dermat. 92, 293—303 (1965).

[30] KLEIN, E., H. L. STOLL, H. A. MILGRAM, H. L. TRAENKLE, R. W. CASE, Y. LAOR, F. HELM, and R. S. NADEL: Tumors of the skin. V. Local administration of anti-tumor agents to multiple superficial basal cell carcinomas. J. invest. Dermat. 45, 489—497 (1965)

[31] FREEMAN, R. G., and J. M. KNOX: Clinical diagnosis of skin tumors by dermatologists. Arch. Dermat. 87, 350 (1963).

[32] STEHLIN, JR., J. S.: Regional chemotherapy for cancers of the skin. In Tumors of the skin. Chicago: Year Book Medical Publishers, Inc. 1964, p. 311.

[33] CREECH, O., and E. T. KREMENTZ: Regional perfusion in melanoma of limbs. J. Amer. med. Ass. 188, 855 (1964).

[34] NICOLLE, F. V., W. H. MATHEWS, and J. D. PALMER: Treatment of malignant melanomas of the skin. J. Amer. med. Ass. 197, 159 (1966).

Chapter 4

Results of Treatment of Skin Cancers

When the results of treatment of skin cancer are analyzed, it is obvious that any of the three methods can be used to achieve a five-year cure rate of 90 per cent or better [1—9]. This is true for both basal cell and squamous cell carcinoma. Since any of these three commonly used methods of treatment, when properly applied, are capable of achieving cure rates of over 90 per cent, the physician can confidently apply the modality most suited to that particular tumor. He also can consider such secondary factors as convenience, expense to the patient, and time for patient and physician. This ability to select the method most suitable for each tumor will result in even higher cure frequencies than if one method is used almost exclusively.

Cancers Analyzed

The tumor types and the modalities used in the treatment of 2,723 tumors in 1,417 patients at Jefferson Davis and Ben Taub General Hospitals and at the Veterans Administration Hospital are shown in Table 1. Charts of patients treated for skin cancer at these hospitals since January 1, 1939, were surveyed. A follow-up of at least one year and a biopsy diagnosis of basal cell or squamous cell carcinoma were pre-requisites. Patients with mucous membrane cancer were not included in this study.

Table 1. *Summary of Experience Treatment Modalities and Tumor Types*

	Basal	Squamous	Total
Curettage and electrodesiccation	1149	649	1798
Surgery	413	249	662
Radiation	156	107	263
Total	1718	1005	2723

Table 2. *Summary of Experience Tumor Size and Treatment Modality*

Treatment	Basal			Squamous		
	< 2 cm.	> 2 cm.	Total	< 2 cm.	> 2 cm.	Total
Curettage and electrodesiccation	1069	80	1149	592	57	649
Surgery	346	67	413	200	449	249
Radiation	128	28	156	84	23	107
Total	1543	175	1718	876	129	1005

Of the 2,723 malignancies, 1,718 were basal cell and 1,005 were squamous cell carcinomas. Treatment was conducted by the respective specialty services of dermatology, surgery and radiology. The procedures were usually performed by the resident physician under staff supervision. Irradiation was used in 263 patients, surgical excision in 662 and curettage and electrodesiccation in 1,798.

All tumors were subdivided by size (larger or smaller than 2 cm. in diameter) and by cell type as shown in Table 2. The anatomic location is shown in Table 3. The number of recurrences among all patients available for follow-up was determined for each tumor type year for five years. Cure rates were then compared.

Table 3. *Anatomic Distribution*

Location	Curettage and electrodesiccation			Surgery			Radiation			Grand total		
	Basal	Squamous	Total	Basal	Squamous	Total	Basal	Squamous	Total	Basal	Squamous	Total
Face	553	282	835	212	100	312	93	67	160	858	449	1307
Nose	304	87	391	87	31	118	39	13	52	430	131	561
Ear	116	65	181	44	44	88	9	9	18	169	118	287
Neck	109	71	180	34	17	51	14	10	24	157	98	255
Hands	7	79	86	9	33	42	—	2	2	16	114	130
Arms	16	39	55	6	8	14	—	4	4	22	51	73
Lower ext.	1	7	8	2	6	8	—	—	—	3	13	16
Trunk	36	10	46	16	5	21	1	—	1	53	15	68
Scalp	3	5	8	3	5	8	—	1	1	6	11	17
Not stated	4	4	8	—	—	—	—	1	1	4	5	9
Total	1149	649	1798	413	249	662	156	107	263	1718	1005	2723

Results with Basal Cell Cancers

With basal cell epitheliomas (Tables 4, 5, 6), five-year cure rates for tumors of all sizes ranged from a low of 95 per cent after surgery to a high of 97.8 per cent after curettage and electrodesiccation. When basal cell carcinomas larger than 2 cm.

Table 4. *Basal Cell Epithelioma Curettage and Electrodesiccation*

	C & D	%	Basal cell epitheliomas C & D < 2 cm.	%	C & D > 2 cm. %	
Total	1149		1069		80	
1 Year	947/948	99.9	880/881	99.9	67/67	100.0
2 Years	753/756	99.6	697/700	99.6	56/56	100.0
3 Years	583/587	99.3	535/539	99.3	48/48	100.0
4 Years	451/457	98.7	414/420	98.6	37/37	100.0
5 Years	311/318	97.8	278/285	97.5	33/33	100.0

Table 5. *Basal Cell Epithelioma Surgical Excision*

	Surgery	%	Basal cell epitheliomas Surgery < 2 cm.	%	Surgery > 2 cn.%	
Total	413		346		67	
1 Year	337/339	99.4	279/281	99.3	58/58	100.0
2 Years	258/262	98.5	215/219	98.2	43/43	100.0
3 Years	211/216	97.7	173/177	97.7	38/39	97.4
4 Years	150/155	96.8	122/125	97.6	28/30	93.3
5 Years	113/119	95.0	90/94	95.7	23/25	92.0

were treated with either surgery or irradiation the cure rate dropped to about 92 per cent. This was not true with curettage and electrodesiccation; however, the perfect

Table 6. *Basal Cell Epithelioma Radiation*

	Radiation	%	Basal cell epithelomias Radiation < 2 cm. %		Radiation > 2 cm. %	
Total	156		128		28	
1 Year	144/144	100.0	120/120	100.0	24/24	100.0
2 Years	128/130	98.5	110/111	99.1	18/19	94.7
3 Years	112/115	97.4	95/97	97.9	17/18	94.4
4 Years	104/107	97.2	92/94	97.9	12/13	92.3
5 Years	93/97	95.9	81/84	96.4	12/13	92.3

treatment record shown in Table 4 for large basal cell epitheliomas reflects a selection of cases. Those large tumors treated by curettage and electrodesiccation were undoubtedly superficial lesions easily amenable to curettage.

By contrast, some of the large lesions treated by surgery or irradiation were quite advanced and would have been difficult to treat by any modality. These presented a major challenge to the therapist. Thus the better results with curettage and electrodesiccation probably reflect selection of cases rather than a superiority of this modality over other forms of treatment. It does indicate, however, that this modality when properly applied is highly effective for treating skin cancers.

Seventeen failures were encountered, seven with curettage and electrodesiccation; six with surgery; and four with radiation. These were recurrences and no metastases occurred in this entire series of 1,718 basal cell epitheliomas.

Results with Squamous Cell Cancers

With squamous cell carcinomas, Tables 7, 8, and 9, the results were quite good with all modalities. The five-year cure rates ranged from 99.5 per cent with curettage

Table 7. *Squamous Cell Carcinoma Curettage and Electrodesiccation*

	C & D	%	Squamous cell carcinomas C & D < 2 cm. %		C & D > 2 cm. %	
Total	649		592		57	
1 Year	545/545	100.0	495/495	100.0	50/50	100.0
2 Years	445/446	99.8	398/399	99.7	47/47	100.0
3 Years	359/359	100.0	317/317	100.0	42/42	100.0
4 Years	275/276	99.6	240/241	99.6	35/35	100.0
5 Years	212/213	99.5	184/185	99.5	28/28	100.0

Table 8. *Squamous Cell Carcinoma Curettage and Electrodesiccation*

	Surgery	%	Squamous cell carcinomas Surgery < 2 cm. %		Surgery > 2 cm. %	
Total	249		200		49	
1 Year	210/211	99.5	167/168	99.4	43/43	100.0
2 Years	154/157	98.1	120/123	97.6	34/34	100.0
3 Years	125/128	97.7	94/97	96.9	31/31	100.0
4 Years	98/102	96.1	72/76	94.7	26/26	100.0
5 Years	77/81	95.1	56/60	93.3	21/21	100.0

and electrodesiccation to 93 per cent for radiation. Surgery yielded a five-year cure rate of 95.1 per cent. Most of the squamous cell carcinomas treated were less than

2 cm. in diameter. Those larger than 2 cm. in diameter were also treated successfully
by all three methods; however, the number of tumors in this category was so small

Table 9. *Squamous Cell Carcinoma Radiation*

	Radiation	%	Squamous cell carcinomas Radiation < 2 cm. %		Radiation > 2 cm. %	
Total	107		84		23	
1 Year	99/101	98.0	79/80	98.8	20/21	95.2
2 Years	96/98	98.0	78/79	98.7	18/19	94.7
3 Years	85/88	96.6	71/73	97.3	14/14	93.3
4 Years	78/83	94.0	66/71	93.0	12/12	100.0
5 Years	69/74	93.2	57/62	91.9	12/12	100.0

that the results probably are not significant. The higher cure rate with curettage and
electrodesiccation again probably reflects a certain selectivity and some of the larger
and more infiltrative lesions were referred for surgery or radiation.

Among the 1,005 patients with squamous cell carcinoma, 368 were followed for
at least five years and of this group, ten had recurrences after treatment. Five of
the ten recurrences were seen after radiation, four after surgery and one after
curettage and electrodesiccation.

These results substantiate that all three treatment modalities are effective when
properly utilized. The figures reported in the accompanying tables in this chapter
should not be compared without keeping in mind that some selection of cases undoubtedly influenced the results. Unusually invasive destructive or sclerosing lesions
were treated by irradiation or by surgery. Certain cases, for example sclerosing
lesions, would not respond satisfactorily to curettage and electrodesiccation and
should be treated by surgical excision. On the other hand, certain lesions should not
be treated by irradiation and in some patients surgery is a poor choice of treatment.
The important conclusion to be derived from these studies, however, is that if the
modalities are properly applied and cases are properly selected for each type of treatment, good results can be obtained.

Table 10. *Summary of Treatment Results all Modalities*

	Basal cell epitheliomas	%	Squamous cell carcinomas	%
Total	1718		1005	
1 Year	1428/1431	99.8	854/857	99.6
2 Years	1139/1148	99.2	695/701	99.1
3 Years	906/918	98.7	569/575	99.0
4 Years	705/719	98.1	451/461	97.8
5 Years	517/534	96.8	358/368	97.3

Most of the tumors treated by all three modalities were less than 2 cm. in diameter
and this indicates that many quite early lesions are being seen. All three methods were
used to treat lesions larger than 2 cm. in diameter and a large diamter does not
necessarily contraindicate the use of curettage and electrodesiccation. Superficial
lesions of large diameter can be destroyed quite easily by this method. In fact it is

Table 11. *Summary of Treatment Results Comparison of Modalities*

	Surgery Squamous & Basal	%	Radiation Squamous & Basal	%	C & D Squamous & Basal	%	Total Squamous & Basal	%
Total	662		263		1798		2723	
1 Year	547/550	99.5	243/245	99.2	1492/1493	99.9	2282/2288	99.7
2 Years	412/419	98.3	224/228	98.2	1198/1202	99.7	1834/1849	99.2
3 Years	336/344	97.7	197/203	97.0	942/946	99.6	1475/1493	98.8
4 Years	248/257	96.5	182/190	95.8	726/733	99.0	1156/1180	98.0
5 Years	190/200	95.0	162/171	94.7	523/531	98.5	875/902	97.0

often preferable for the superficial lesion since destruction can be accomplished and healing will follow with a good cosmetic result and without skin grafting or other reconstructive procedures. If curettage and electrodesiccation is used judiciously in superficial lesions, the cure frequency is as good as with any other modality.

References

[1] PATERSON, R., M. TOD, and M. RUSSELL: The results of radium and X-ray therapy in malignant disease. Second Statistical Report from the Holt Radium Inst., Manchester, Edinburgh: E. & S. Livingstone, Ltd. 1946.

[2] EBERHARD, T. P.: Treatment of epitheliomas of the skin. Radiology 49, 620—627 (1947).

[3] WARD, G. E., and J. W. HENDRICK: Malignant epithelial tumors of the skin of head and neck. Amer. J. Surg. 79, 711 (1950).

[4] MACOMBER, W. B., M. K. H. WANG, and J. G. SULLIVAN: Cutaneous epithelioma: A Study of 853 lesions. Plast. reconstr. Surg. 24, 545—562 (1959).

[5] FERRARA, R. J.: The private dermatologist and skin cancer: Clinic study of 226 epitheliomas derived from five dermatologic practices. Arch. Dermat. 81, 225—234 (1960).

[6] KNOX, J. M., T. W. LYLES, E. W. SHAPIRO, and R. D. MARTIN: Curettage and electrodesiccation in treatment of skin cancer. Arch. Dermat. 82, 197—204 (1960).

[7] WILLIAMSON, G. S., and R. JACKSON: Treatment of basal cell carcinoma by electrodesiccation and curettage. Canad. med. Assoc. J. 86, 855 (1962).

[8] SWEET, R. D.: The treatment of basal cell carcinoma by curettage. Brit. J. Dermat. 75, 137—158 (1963).

[9] SIMPSON, J. R.: The treatment of rodent ulcers by curettage and cauterization. Brit. J. Derm. 78, 147—148 (1966).

Chapter 5

Treatment of Precancerous Dermatoses

In addition to wrinkling and degeneration, sun exposure produces premalignant conditions that may eventuate in skin cancer. Included among the precancerous dermatoses are certain types of keratoses, cutaneous horn and leukoplakia. The premalignant keratoses are actinic (senile), arsenical and post-irradiation keratoses. Cutaneous horn usually begins as a hyperkeratotic actinic keratosis and, like any other actinic keratosis, may evolve into a squamous cell carcinoma. Leukoplakia, which by definition is limited to mucous membranes, is closely related to actinic keratosis.

The main microscopic feature common to the premalignant dermatoses is malignant dyskeratosis – a disruption in the maturation of epidermal cells manifested by nuclear variation, an increase in the ratio of nucleus to cytoplasm, and individual cell keratinization. Lesions clinically appearing larger, thicker and more infiltrative are usually the most advanced microscopically as well, although ulceration, infection, hyperkeratosis and other secondary changes may be misleading. Some of these lesions remain benign and non-invasive for years, but approximately 20 per cent eventually invade the dermis as squamous cell carcinomas.

Actinic (Senile) keratoses develop almost exclusively on areas exposed to sunlight – the face, neck, ears, hands and arms. The incidence is proportional to the total amount of exposure and inversely proportional to the amount of pigment. Fair-skinned people working outdoors in a region of intense sunshine are more predisposed to actinic keratoses. Such people can protect themselves by avoiding unnecessary exposure and properly using clothing and sunscreens. A broad-brimmed hat and long-sleeved garments should be worn. An excellent sunscreen is 10 per cent para-aminobenzoic acid in vanishing cream. Red veterinary petrolatum also is effective and cosmetically acceptable. A variety of commercially available preparations are effective.

Early keratoses often can be managed conservatively. Involved areas should be lubricated three to four times a day with petrolatum or another good lubricant. Individual lesions may be treated with weekly applications of 20 per cent podophyllin in tincture of benzoin or destroyed by freezing with liquid nitrogen or dry ice. Trichloracetic acid (50 per cent) also is effective. A hydrophilic ointment containing 5 per cent 5-fluorouracil may also be used.

Advanced keratoses must be completely destroyed before they undergo malignant change into squamous cell carcinoma. A biopsy specimen should be obtained. The most acceptable methods of treatment are 1) curettage followed by electrodesiccation, and 2) surgical excision. These technics are discussed more fully elsewhere in this chapter. Burks and others have shown that dermabrasion can improve actinically damaged skin and retard the development of new actinic keratoses.

Post-irradiation and arsenical keratoses: Physicians should use ionizing irradiation cautiously and conservatively and only when other safe treatments prove ineffective. The physician and patient must be adequately protected when using radiation therapy. Fortunately, post-irradiation keratoses are becoming less common.

Excessive ingestion of inorganic arsenic also can cause keratoses. Prescribing inorganic arsenic is rarely justified but such a prescription should be marked "non-refillable".

Treatment is identical to that outlined for actinic keratoses. However, when severe chronic radiodermatitis accompanies keratoses, treatment may be more difficult and necessitate skin grafting.

Early leukoplakia of the lips and mouth may occasionally be eliminated through conservative and prophylactic measures. Use of tabacco in all forms should be discontinued. Dental abnormalities should be corrected and dental hygiene must be excellent. Any source of irritation, including strong tooth paste and mouth rinses, should be eliminated. Vitamin A (Vi-Dom-A buccal tablets 75,000 to 150,000 units daily) may be of value. If the lips are involved, dryness can be avoided and protection provided by using A-Fil Sunstick. Lipstick also provides good protection.

Advanced leukoplakia requires more vigorous treatment. Carcinoma frequently develops in advanced leukoplakia, and cancer of the mouth carries a serious prognosis. All measures recommended for early lesions should be instituted and if there is erosion, ulceration, fissuring, or pronounced thickening in any of the involved sites, a biopsy is indicated to rule out actual malignancy. All advanced lesions should be destroyed by curettage and electrodesiccation or by excision.

Chapter 6

Prevention

General Measures

The major cause of skin cancer is sunlight and this is the logical place to consider a preventive attack. Although complete avoidance of sun exposure eliminates the danger of sun-induced skin cancer, this measure is neither feasible nor acceptable. Sunlight has beneficial effects, for example vitamin D synthesis, so that complete avoidance of the sun is not desirable except possibly for the rare unfortunate person with xeroderma pigmentosa or for one with exquisite sensitivity to sunlight who is almost certainly doomed to an early cancer death.

Furthermore this type of preventive attack is hampered by the fact that most people already have received substantial doses of ultraviolet light in childhood before they are seen by the doctor or before they become aware of any danger of sunlight. Significant actinic skin damage is observed even in young adults in their 20's [1]. On the other hand, cancer patients often develop few cancers in the winter or when they protect their skin and there is some evidence that these actinic changes may be reversible [2].

Thus a sensible attitude toward sunlight exposure is to avoid unnecessary exposure and to dress properly with a hat, sun glasses and longsleeved garments when in the sunlight. Persons unusually sensitive to sun, for example albinos and fair-complexioned persons, must be especially cautious. They should be discouraged from outdoor recreational pursuits such as golf, boating and tennis, particularly if their occupation requires them to be outdoors. People with dark complexions also should protect themselves if exposed a great deal during their regular working day. Moderate amounts of pigment afford only partial protection and large cumulative doses can produce skin damage and cancer even in dark-skinned Caucasians. All these precautions are more urgent in latitudes near the tropics and in regions having hot and sunny climates.

Unfortunately "sun fadism" still prompts many people to expose themselves excessively to the sun, and physicians should use every opportunity to emphasize the fallacy and danger of this fad. It would be well to extend this warning to children and young adults since these age groups will benefit most by preventive measures.

Topical Measures

Topical unctions, usually oils, have been used with sun exposure in the past and are still being used. Most common among these are mineral or vegetable oils and white petrolatum. These afford some protection but not nearly enough in most climates. White petrolatum affords protection equivalent to about four times the M.E.D. [3]. The M.E.D. at mid-day of summer in Texas is about 10 to 15 minutes; therefore white petrolatum protects for about 40—60 minutes, an inadequate amount for most outdoor activities in this climate.

Adding a variety of agents to an ointment effectively increases its screening ability. Some substances, for example talc and titanium dioxide, act as opaque shields to light. Their effectiveness is apparent in the well-preserved skin of women who habitually wear make-up. Several families of compounds — para-aminobenzoates, anthranilates, salicylates, cinnamates, benzophenones—have been used as ultraviolet absorbers to enhance the screening effect of topical sunscreen preparations. Although many of these compounds have been added to commercials unscreen preparations, the protection given by more than 50 of these preparations is only about four to ten times M.E.D., i. e. approximately 60 to 150 minutes' protection in Texas in July.

More effective sunscreens can be prepared easily. ROTHMAN [4] demonstrated that 15 per cent PABA in Ruggles cream is 50 to 100 times as effective as the vehicle alone. Ten per cent PABA in vanishing cream and several benzophenones and acrylonitriles are effective in the laboratory in the range of 50 to 100 times the M.E.D. [3, 5]. It is hoped that highly effective preparations will soon be ready for commercial distribution. Another preparation now available, red veterinary petrolatum, is equally effective and cosmetically reasonably acceptable [6]. While most commercially available compounds absorb only mid-ultraviolet wavelengths, the benzophenones absorb both mid and long ultraviolet wavelengths and thus may be more effective in people with photosensitivity to long ultraviolet [7].

Patients should be encouraged to use an effective sunscreen regularly before participating in any outdoor activity involving sun exposure. To prevent wrinkling, cutaneous degeneration and skin cancer, regular use of a sunscreen idally should begin in childhood. With exposure early in life, this time-dosage relationship increases likelihood of skin cancer with lower total cumulative exposure in adult life. Intense exposure early in life also seriously restricts the amount of exposure advisable in adult years at a time when occupation may require being outdoors for extended periods.

Systemic Measures

Only recently have systemic means of preventing skin cancer been seriously investigated. It was encouraging to find a significant protective effect in a double-blind study in which 250 mg. of chloroquine was given daily to skin cancer patients [8]. Results of this clinical study are supported by finding fewer experimentally-induced skin tumors in mice fed chloroquine in their laboratory chow [9]. Unfortunately, the use of chloroquine must be curtailed because of its association with possibly irreversible retinal damage [10]. However, the demonstration of an appreciable protective effect by a systemically administered agent is intriguing and indicates that safer drugs almost certainly will be discovered.

In an extensive clinical trial, psoralen was not an effective preventive [*11, 12*]. In fact, experimental studies with animals indicate that prolonged systemic use of psoralens and intense ultraviolet may produce ocular cataracts and an increased frequency of skin cancers [*13, 14*]. However, these animals received higher doses of psoralen and ultraviolet than have been given to man. There is no evidence that ocular damage has occurred in men given therapeutic doses.

References

[*1*] COCKERELL, E. G., R. G. FREEMAN, and J. M. KNOX: Changes after prolonged exposure to sunlight. Arch. Dermat. **84**, 467—472 (1961).

[*2*] GERSTEIN, W., and R. G. FREEMAN: Transplantation of actinically damaged skin. J. invest. Dermat. **39**, 295—298 (1962).

[*3*] ROSSMAN, R. E., J. M. KNOX, and R. G. FREEMAN: Acrylonitriles: A new group of ultraviolet absorbing compounds. J. invest. Dermat. **39**, 449—453 (1962).

[*4*] ROTHMAN, S., and A. B. HENNINGSEN: The sunburn protecting effect of para-aminobenzoic acid. J. invest. Dermat. **9**, 307 (1947).

[*5*] KNOX, J. M.: Ultraviolet absorbers. J. Soc. Cos. Chemists **13**, 119—124 (1962).

[*6*] MACEACHERN, W. N., and O. F. JILLSON: A practical sunscreen—"Red Vet Pet". Arch. Dermat. **89**, 147—150 (1964).

[*7*] KNOX, J. M., J. D. GUIN, and E. G. COCKERELL: Benzophenones. Ultraviolet light absorbing agents. J. invest. Dermat. **29**, 435—444 (1957).

[*8*] GUIN, J. D., and J. M. KNOX: The effect of systemic chloroquine therapy on actinic keratoses. Arch. Dermat. **80**, 347—348 (1959).

[*9*] KNOX, J. M., A. C. GRIFFIN, and R. E. HAKIM: Effect of chloroquine on erythematous and carcinogenic response to ultraviolet light. Arch. Dermat. **81**, 570—576 (1961).

[*10*] —, and D. W. OWENS: The chloroquine mystery. Submitted for publication.

[*11*] MACDONALD, E. J., A. C. GRIFFIN, C. E. HOPKINS, L. SMITH, H. GARRETT, and G. L. BLACK: Psoralen prophylaxis against skin cancer. Report of clinical trial. I. J. invest. Dermat. **41**, 213—217 (1963).

[*12*] HOPKINS, C. E., J. C. BELISARIO, E. J. MACDONALD, and C. T. DAVIS: Psoralen prophylaxis against skin cancer. Report of clinical trial. II. J. invest. Dermat. **41**, 219—223 (1963).

[*13*] GRIFFIN, A. C., R. E. HAKIM, and J. M. KNOX: The wave length effect upon erythemal and carcinogenic response in psoralen treated mice. J. invest. Dermat. **31**, 289—295 (1958).

[*14*] CLOUD, T. M.: Photosensitization of eye with methoxsalen. II. Chronic effects. Arch. Ophth. **66**, 689 (1961).

Subject Index

Monographs already published

SCHINDLER, R., Lausanne: Die tierische Zelle in Zellkultur (Volume 1).

Neuroblastomas — Biochemical Studies. Edited by C. BOHUON, Villejuif (Volume 2, Symposium).

HUEPER, W. C., Bethesda: Occupational and Environmental Cancers of the Respiratory System (Volume 3).

GOLDMAN, L., Cincinnati: Laser Cancer Research (Volume 4).

METCALF, D., Melbourne: The Thymus. Its Role in Immune Responses, Leukaemia Development and Carcinogenesis (Volume 5).

Malignant Transformation by Viruses. Edited by W. H. KIRSTEN, Chicago (Volume 6, Symposium).

MOERTEL, CH. G., Rochester: Multiple Primary Malignant Neoplasms. Their Incidence and Significance (Volume 7).

New Trends in the Treatment of Cancer. Edited by L. MANUILA, S. MOLES and P. RENTCHNICK, Genève (Volume 8).

LINDENMANN, J., Zürich / P. A. KLEIN, Gainesville, Florida: Immunological Aspects of Viral Oncolysis (Volume 9).

NELSON, R. S., Houston: Radioactive Phosphorus in the Diagnosis of Gastrointestinal Cancer (Volume 10).

FREEMANN, R. G., and J. M. KNOX, Houston: Treatment of Skin Cancer (Volume 11).

In production

LYNCH, H. T., Omaha: Hereditary Factors in Carcinoma (Vol. 12).

MARSDEN, H. B., and J. K. STEWARD, Manchester: Tumours in Children (Vol. 13).

In preparation

ANGLESIO, E., Torino: The Treatment of Hodgkin's Disease.

CHIAPPA, S., Milano: Endolymphatic Radiotherapy in Malignant Lymphomas.

DENOIX, P., Villejuif: Le traitement des cancers du sein.

FISHER, E. R., Pittsburgh: Ultrastructure of Human Normal and Neoplastic Prostate.

FUCHS, W. A., Bern: Lymphography and Tumordiagnosis.

GRUNDMANN, E., Wuppertal-Elberfeld: Morphologie und Cytochemie der Carcinogenese.

HAYWARD, J. L., London: Cancer of the Breast: Hormonal Changes.

IRLIN, I. S., Moskva: Mechanisms of Viral Carcinogenesis.

KERN, G., Köln: Carcinoma in situ.

KOLDOVSKY, P., Praha: Transplantation Tumor Specific Antigen (TTSA).

LANGLEY, F. A., Manchester: Epithelial Abnormalities of the Cervix Uteri.

MARTZ, G., Zürich: Hormonbehandlung der Tumoren.

MATHÉ, G., Villejuif: L'Immunotherapie des cancer.

MEEK, E. S., Bristol: Antiviral and Antitumour Agents of Biological Origin.

NEWMAN, M. K., Detroit: Neuropathies and Myopathies Associated with Occult Malignancies.

ODARTCHENKO, N., Lausanne: Prolifération cellulaire érythropiétique.

PACK, G. T., New York: Clinical Aspects of Cancer Immunity and Cancer Susceptibility.

PACK, G. T., New York / A. H. ISLAMI, New York: Tumors of the Liver.

RITZMAN, S. E., Galveston / W. C. LEVIN, Galveston: The Syndrome of Macroglobulinemia.

ROY-BURMAN, P., Los Angeles: Biochemical Mechanisms Involved in the Inhibition of Metabolic Processes by Purine, Pyramidine, and Nucleoside Analogs.

SOKOLOFF, B., Lakeland/Florida: Cancer and Serotonin.

WEIL, R., Lausanne: Biological and Structural Properties of Polyoma Virus and its DNA.

WILLIAMS, D. C., Caterham, Surrey: The Basis for Therapy of Hormon Sensitive Tumours.

WILLIAMS, D. C., Caterham, Surrey: The Biochemistry of Metastasis.

ZILBER, L. A., Moskva: Virogenetic Theory of Cancer Origin.

Herstellung: Konrad Triltsch, Graphischer Betrieb, Würzburg